EAT & GROW SLIM *FOR GOOD!*

The Montignac Slimming Sensation

to lose 19 pounds in 2 weeks

incorporating

The foods that make you lose weight

The Montignac Slimming Sensation
to lose 19 pounds in 2 weeks
incorporating
The foods that make you lose weight

Published MMII by The Windsor Group
The Old School House, St John's Court,
Moulsham Street, Chelmsford,
Essex CM2 0JD

ISBN 1-903904-20-X

Table of Contents

Part One

Reach Your Ideal Weight Without Hunger
or
Eat and Stay Slim

What is the Montignac Method?

To put it as simply as possible: it is an effective and safe opportunity to reach your desired weight, the principle being: 'Eat and lose weight at the same time!' Imagine looking in the mirror, or getting on the scales in the morning and the self-critical moment as you choose what to wear: How do you feel? Good or not so good? Perhaps a kilo or more lighter? But how?

Now there is an eating method where you can become slim through eating. So you can be your ideal weight without starving, without giving up too much, without an all too tedious diet? You are dreaming, aren't you?

Well, a dream can become reality.

The dream of losing weight, just through eating, can come true for you straightaway – if you want. It all depends on you; you will:

- lose weight
- reach your ideal weight
- stay slim and active

How? At any rate, not by going hungry, or by tedious calorie counting, self-denial or excessive sacrifices. On the contrary! A purposeful and informed way of eating is not only fun but also healthy and vital.

But let us be honest: anyone who has weight problems will first try a conventional diet, of which there are loads. There are basically hardly any differences between most diets. They are based on two principles:

- to reduce energy intake – usually fats
- do some sport

Unfortunately the results are anything but gratifying, as not only statistics but also numerous examples of personal experience demonstrate – we've all heard: 'I've already tried lots of diets and I'm just starting a new one...'

There is something wrong or at least very dubious about this. There must be a better way of sorting out your weight without having to make your way laboriously from one diet to another.

By chance Michel Montignac came across some statistical investigations into diabetes, according to which 80% of all diabetics are obese. It seemed possible that both ailments had the same origin.

What is the basic cause here?

Weight loss occurs when you eat food with a low glycaemic index. With diabetics of type II who were suffering from hyperinsulinism this was actually successful and led to an improvement in their diabetes. It was therefore enough to apply the dietetic principle 'consume carbohydrates with a low glycaemic index', test it and find that the principle was successful.

In order to be really successful in losing weight without starving the only thing you have to do is to select the right foods without limiting quantities or doing any extra sport.

But to be really successful you also have to pursue the following goals. We must:

⇧ demystify traditional ideas with sufficiently convincing arguments so that we can abandon them once and for all

⇧ provide a scientific basis which is essential for the understanding of the metabolic processes involved in weight gain

⇧ establish simple rules and give scientific reasons for them

⇧ think about all the possible ways of applying this method down to the smallest detail

⇧ develop a method which will also act as a practical adviser

One thing should be made clear right from the start. It is utterly wrong to assume that we put weight on because we eat too much. We put weight on because we eat the wrong things.

We must therefore learn:

⇧ to eat properly

⇧ to deal with our food supply in a careful way; in other words, to organise our food intake with awareness and control

As we do this we will discover that straightaway we will be able to harmonise our family, social and business interests and obligations with our personal pleasure in food, without putting on weight.

In addition we will learn to eat in a healthier way that will nevertheless be enjoyable and satisfying.

There will be no diet put forward here: quite the opposite. A diet always has the disadvantage that at some point it ends and we can then revert to the old routine.

The Montignac Method is a way of eating which is scientifically supported. With this method you learn how to maintain your weight without renouncing the pleasures of the table. This method not only works at home but on week-days at work, when you're with friends or in the restaurant.

At the same time you will be amazed to discover that, as you put into prac-tice the nutritional principles that are recommended here, you will regain your physical and emotional vitality. Why is that so? Certain eating habits are very often the reason why we are tired and have less energy for the de-mands made by sport or work. Yet with a few changes in our food this dam-age to our efficiency will be prevented. This means no longer being tired after meals, being able to achieve more, being livelier and more energetic.

Learning this method and applying it will pay off in terms of good all-round health.

The advantage is obvious: you will discover new energy – which you have always had lying dormant, but which you can now awaken. You will simply get on better at work and at home. Moreover, the gastro-intestinal complaints that often accompany overweight will disappear. Your digestive system will find a new balance.

You can achieve all this if you are willing to live with this new, effective method a while you will be able to convince yourself. After all, why should you believe in something until you understand it and can confirm it through your own experience?

Obesity is a part of nature's plan

The phenomenon of obesity is not found in nature. In the animal world no signs of it can be found, except among household pets. But there are other reasons for that.

In so-called 'primitive' cultures the phenomenon of obesity occurred rarely or not at all. It was early later that some cultures began to worship or admire those who were particularly fat. But this was generally in societies where food was in short supply. Therefore only the very wealthy could afford to accumulate fat.

But the reason they were fat was not because they had eaten more – although that was certainly true in some cases – but because they mainly ate different-ly.

Today we live in a completely different world. Everyone can be fat today, have his 'very own' layer of fat without having to be rich or be deserving of special worship. Exceptions are Japanese Sumo wrestlers or weight lifters and perhaps all-in wrestlers as well. For the rest, however, the view is that excessive weight is neither desirable nor worthwhile nor advantageous in any way. However, that doesn't mean that we must now all become as slim as a reed. Rather it means that obesity is not destiny or fate but can be changed.

And so this is what matters.

Change your weight with awareness!

Let us look at the USA. Sixty-five percent of all Americans are too fat. Thirty three percent are obese.

A glance back into history tells us that obesity is a so-called illness caused by civilisation. We know it from Ancient Rome and from Egypt as well.

Are we prepared to put up with this? Or do we want to do something about it!

If you ask a so-called specialist why you are overweight when you eat almost nothing, he will wager that it's down to heredity or predisposition.

If we consult a nutritional expert and put his method into practice but without having very much success, he will attribute the blame to us, perhaps to our lack of will power or that famous hereditary predisposition.

A certain hereditary proneness to overweight is, of course, not to be denied. To make heredity responsible for everything, however, would be fatalistic and wrong. Human beings hold their fate in their own hands, at least to a certain extent.

Once again, in the USA a hundred years ago obesity was unknown. Today, a hundred years later, it exists. Heredity? Who is supposed to have passed it on? Heredity and inherited tendencies can be ruled out. What remains are bad eating habits.

Bad eating habits are to blame for obesity

This also means that – like every other habit – we can change them. This is not an inborn but an acquired phenomenon, and therefore it can be changed!

We have already mentioned another argument for being fat: you eat a lot or just too much. Excessive eating ('hyperphagia') is the reason accepted by specialists for obesity. People are fat because they eat too much.

Unfortunately, that's not exactly true.

As a counter-argument you definitely know someone who eats a great deal at any time, no matter how inconvenient, and yet who is not fat at all, who is even perhaps extremely thin.

If you ask obese people about their eating habits you will find that their calorie intake is extremely low. This contradiction can be explained by the fact that the fatter people are, the more desperately calories matter.

We are amazed by the massive amount of food consumed by our parents and grandparents on social occasions in the past. Compared to them we eat far less today, something by the way that has long been proved.

The reason people were able to eat more in the past is often explained by the fact that they exerted themselves more physically. They walked when they went anywhere, they performed hard physical labour, had to climb many stairs instead of using a lift and lived in houses with little heating.

This situation is not typical of all levels of the population, however. Incidentally, of course, they also sat for long periods just as we do today, especially when they were on a journey, in the past in a carriage, today in a traffic jam.

In spite of all that, there were, of course, still obese people, but it was not a widespread social phenomenon as it is today.

Even mentioning the cold or central heating is not a convincing argument. In the past people had more clothes and were wrapped up more warmly, even in the summer.

So, to sum up: our ancestors were not less fat because they used up more energy. The generally increasing incidence of obesity has other causes, which we must look for first in the deterioration of our eating habits.

It is our incorrect eating habits and also the constant use of low-calorie diets and foods which determine our modern way of eating and which are responsible for obesity. They are the cause – and thus they can be changed!

We must change the way we eat

Our new philosophy of life is not that less is more – in old language: calorie counting provides no advantages – except in that we are eating sensibly and mindfully. Armed with the knowledge of some food-specific facts, we are in the position to shed our excessive weight for ever and to do it not by starving ourselves but by EATING!

Away with counting calories
The calorie myth

Something to think about. . .

In order to change our eating habits in a positive and long-lasting way we need to not only think about these habits but also to know where they come from. It is therefore important for us to know how we have actually arrived at our present-day attitudes to food, for it is only what we know that we can change.

For this reason we would like to take another little detour into our recent past to see how our thoughts and ideas about nutrition have changed. The reason this is helpful is because even today we are still confronted with yesterday's arguments!

Cultural and social conditions have changed decisively in the last 50 years. In the past, food was the 'source of life'. Everyone was convinced that the way they ate had a direct effect on their state of mind and that food was 'the best medicine', as Hippocrates put it as long ago as 500BC.

Food was so important then because it was scarce and expensive. A few decades ago the nightmare visions of famines, deprivation and shortages were still present in people's minds.

In contrast today our shopping baskets are filled to overflowing. Food plays such an unimportant role that the wastefulness shown by most of our contemporaries is really more than insulting in the face of numerous starving people worldwide. Moreover, in the interests of a flourishing economy food is destroyed instead of being used elsewhere. This is how far we have progressed.

We no longer earn our bread through the sweat of our brow, nor are leftovers saved and put to good use. They end up in the rubbish bin; they're disposed of, end of story.

Something decisive must have happened for such a lack of respect for food to have developed gradually. This is nothing other than the existing surplus of foodstuffs. This surplus, which came about as a result of the drastic changes in the food industry at the end of the Second World War, has led to a debasement of our 'daily bread' and above all has changed the way we basically think.

After 1945 our society had to deal with two main problems: on the one hand there was the great increase in population resulting from the post-war baby boom and the arrival of thousands of refugees; on the other hand cities grew as a result of the rise in population and the increasing migration from the land.

It was absolutely vital to produce food in greater quantities and, to a large extent, in a different way, because for the first time in the history of mankind the areas where food was grown were all at once no longer the same as the areas where it was eaten.

In 1950 80% of the food consumed by a small town was produced within a radius of 50 kilometres. The remaining 20% came from the surrounding countryside or from other countries.

Today this ratio is completely the other way around.

When foodstuffs were still processed on the spot the resulting waste was used as fertiliser. From the time when people began to export foodstuffs, nothing could be utilised in this way any more, so people were forced to fall back on other methods of fertilisation.

In the last 50 years, as a result of numerous increasingly efficient technologies, the food industry has continued to develop. These far-reaching changes have had several repercussions.

⇨ They led to a considerable **rise in yields** through:

- mechanisation
- the massive use of artificial fertiliser
- the increasing use of pesticides, insecticides and fungicides
- the introduction of intensive livestock farming

⇨ They led to the development of new **conservation techniques** through:

- the spread of refrigeration and freezer processes
- the use of additives and other chemical methods of conservation

The result of all these measures was extremely impressive and exceeded all expectations. From this time on there was a part of mankind who lived as if there was an abundance of food that they would never need to worry about again.

And yet. . . Very early on it was established that there were often excessive weight gains. Solutions were sought and scientists produced solutions. Their hypotheses were basically as follows.

Because body weight increased greatly when there was an abundance of food available, it seems reasonable to suppose that these two things are connected.

It was therefore assumed that the human body functions rather like the boiler of a steam engine. To live, this boiler needs energy, which it gets through the supply of food (energy supply). On the other hand it also uses up energy (energy consumption). Overweight can therefore only be the result of an imbalance between energy supply and energy consumption. Through this imbalance the additional pounds become an energy store.

All in all, this means that there has either been an energy supply that is too large or an energy consumption that is too small. If someone is overweight, it is because they have either eaten too much or had too little physical exercise or both at the same time. We should all be very familiar with this kind of thinking, but it does not correspond with reality.

Regardless, what has developed from this is the nutritional theory of calorie reduction. Since energy supply was expressed in calorie units, people were put in the position where they divided all foods according to their calorie content, on the basis of their weight and composition (carbohydrates, fats, proteins). Yet right from the beginning this method was full of errors. You kept a close eye on your calorie intake but did not consider, for example, what was happening with your digestive system.

Conventional, restrictively structured dietetics, which is based on a method of calorie reduction, developed from this.

When dietetics fixed a person's daily energy requirements at about 2,500 calories, the explanation given for this was that body weight could be influenced by the actual calorific intake in either direction.

When, therefore, you consume 3,000 calories a day, there will be a surplus of 500 calories which is stored in the body and, logically, will result in a certain increase in weight.

If, on the other hand, you get by on only 2,000 calories, there will be a deficit of 500 calories which will make the body draw on its fat reserves to even out the difference. As a result, there would logically be a reduction in weight.

The calorie theory therefore says that, to lose weight, you only need to eat less and that if you put on weight, you are eating too much.

In the last few decades this over-simplified plan, based on a naïve starting-point, was the most important for dietetics. Unfortunately, it is still officially propagated in the nutrition departments of hospitals and taught in Schools of Dietetics. Yet whoever takes the calorie method as a basis, as most dietetic specialists still do, ignores the following:

The measures taken by our body to adapt and to regulate.

Human beings are not machines and they do not function in a mechanical way. This assumption that human beings function like machines – and the observations above suggest this way of thinking – does not take individual peculiarities and characteristics into consideration.

Every human being is a unique creature. We must take this into account where nutrition is concerned as well.

In addition, the viewpoint described above confuses quantity with quality. It is not just a matter of how much you eat, but what you eat as well as attitude towards it.

Unlike the conventional view, an obese person is not necessarily someone who eats too much. In most cases the opposite is true. Let us take France as an example. (We can observe something similar in other countries too). This shows us that in France

- only 15% of obese people eat too much (2,800–4,000 calories)
- 35% of obese people eat normally (2,000–2,700 calories)
- 50% of obese people eat less (800–1,500 calories)

Among professional sportsmen and women it has been found that a constant body weight can be maintained with an intake of between 2,500 and 9,000 calories; this does not depend on the type of sport **they do** but on the constitution of the individual.

With an intake of just 2,000 calories a day the marathon runner Alain Mimoun maintained his weight and successfully completed his tough training, whereas the racing cyclist Jacques Anquetil needed 6,000 calories to maintain his weight and to keep in form.

Although medical literature is strangely reserved on this subject, a great number of such investigations were published. They show that calorie intake has no influence on whether you are fat, thin or have a normal weight. There is no significant connection between overweight and calorie intake.

Now let us leave France and take ourselves across the pond to the USA.

For 45 years (!) 89 million (!) Americans have constantly followed a reduced-calorie eating plan. The calorie is always with us. Through advertising and the media it is firmly fixed in the American consciousness. (But even European countries are up there with them in their attitude to the calorie.) Alongside all the calorie counting they are scrupulously careful to take a lot of exercise to make absolutely sure they don't consume a single calorie more than necessary.

And are they successful?

Statistics show us a shattering result.

Although more than a third of the population consistently uses the calorie-controlled method of dieting and exercise intensively every day, weight is still gained. Or in figures: two-thirds of the population today are overweight and 33% are obese.

The easiest way to understand why the calorie-controlled method of eating, which has been promoted for over 40 years, is marked by a lack of success is to look at the example of America. Unfortunately, many European countries, especially Germany, are following in their footsteps.

Here are an additional couple of arguments, which show that calorie counting is still very theoretical and absolutely inaccurate.

- If you compare the details of the various calorie charts you will find that they differ greatly from one another.
- The calorie content of foods varies according to whether they are eaten raw or cooked (with fats or without).
- The amount of fat (which can alter the calorie content considerably) can differ greatly from one piece of meat to another. It depends on how the animal was reared and how the meat was prepared.
- The (theoretical) calculation of calories never takes into account the conditions by which fats and carbohydrates are absorbed in the small intestine. The absorption will vary depending on the fibre content of the food eaten at the same meal.
- If the food contains a great deal of fibre (especially soluble fibre) absorption of the so-called calories can be decisively reduced.
- L. Fakambi's work has shown that fermented cheese (Gruyere, other Swiss cheese) contains a large amount of calcium, which binds with the non-absorbed fats. The associated calories will be excreted.
- The 'type' of calories one consumes influences the way they will be used. Saturated fats are easier to store, while polyunsaturated fats (especially omega-3 fatty acids) are easier to use and so can be burnt off.
- Finally, simply counting calories does not take into account the time when food will be eaten. It has been found that the absorption of carbohydrates, fats and proteins varies according to the time of day, or even the season (chronobiology). This absorption also depends on the chemical conditions found by the food in the gut. This environment is influenced by the food's properties, the order in which it has reached the gut and how much of it there is.

This leads us to the conclusion that it is pointless to count calories without including these additional criteria.

Something else to think about: Figure 1 shows that the continuous use of low calorie diets will end up making the body resistant to weight loss – in other words obese. With a decreasing number of calories, the diet will become less and less effective and the body will not only return to its original weight but also will lay down extra fat reserves.

Figure 1 A life of misery for the overweight but 'undernourished'.

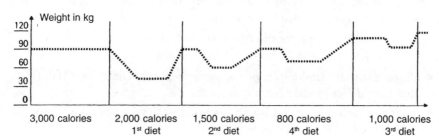

Unfortunately, the calorie theory has been widely circulated among the general public, because it is believed to have a genuine scientific basis. It has been so widely accepted and fixed in people's minds that there is hardly any canteen, cafeteria or canteen kitchen where the calorie content for each dish is not given so that their customers can 'know' what they're eating.

Hardly a week goes by without one of the many magazines around devoting its front page to the subject of diet and calorie meals, compiled by a team of nutritionists. Complying with the calorie theory and exaggerating just a little, they recommend us to eat 'a mandarin orange for breakfast, half a rusk at 11 o'clock, one chickpea for lunch and an olive in the evening...'

There are cookery books that work out precise calorie counts for their recipes: 156 calories... no more and no less. Don't you think that's strange? You might almost say it's unintentionally amusing to use such precision with such an imprecise method.

But after all, as we take this line of reasoning further, who is prepared to admit that they've made a mistake in the last few years or that that they've been duped by a mistake – or rather a mistaken belief?

Nevertheless, we have to ask ourselves how this fallacious calorie theory has lasted so long. One answer is that reduced calorie diets very often have results. Doing without food – the basis of these diets – inevitably leads to a certain amount of weight loss.

But as we have seen, this is only ever a temporary result. Sooner or later you don't just weigh as much as you did before the diet, you usually weigh even more. Another answer is that 'low calorie' as a concept is an enormous economic factor, from which a pressure group of representatives from the food industry and some misguided cooks and nutritionists make a profit.

On the wrong track
A warning about reduced calorie diets

We have already shown how the concept of 'balance' between energy intake and energy consumption in the human body came about in the past and how the reduced calorie method of dieting – seen to be ineffective – developed.

It seems to be a paradox that the more you count calories and eat in a calorie-conscious way, the harder it is not just to lose weight but to maintain your weight. There's some success at the beginning, but in the long run it's a laborious and exhausting undertaking.

Anyone who has ever been on a diet can confirm this. Often when you get on the scales afterwards, you weigh more than you did before.

Why is that?

As an example, let's take someone who eats about 2,500 calories a day and who is a few pounds overweight. If they reduce their intake to 2,000 calories, according to the low calorie method, there will be a shortfall of 500 calories, so they should lose weight. But the body, which has become accustomed to an intake of 2,500 calories, makes up the missing 500 calories from its fat, which leads to a corresponding weight loss. So far, so good.

After a short time, which can vary considerably depending on the individual, it becomes clear that no more weight is being lost, in spite of the fact that there has been no interruption to the diet; in fact, it has been strictly followed.

More is less

What has happened? Quite simply, the body has become accustomed to an intake of 2,000 calories and reacts by slowing down its metabolism. If you decide to carry on with the diet after a short break, hoping to lose weight again, you will be in for a disappointment: instead of losing weight you will put it on! The explanation is extremely simple.

The human body is driven by a survival instinct, which is aroused when there is a shortage of food or, rather, of energy. Since there was an earlier reduction in calorie intake, which the body has adjusted to by consuming less energy, this instinct to survive has caused the body to reduce its energy consumption still further. This means that the daily calorie requirement has dropped to 1,700 calories, for example, so that new reserves can be laid down.

We mustn't forget either that the human body has not changed in its habits as quickly as the human brain has. The body is still living in the past, when hunger and deprivation were well known. These memories are present in our subconscious and this behaviour brings them back to life.

The human body is guided by the same survival instinct as, say, that of a dog, who will bury its supply of bones when it is very hungry. Strangely, the instinct to lay down supplies is only aroused in an animal when it's hungry.

When the body experiences a shortage, i.e. when there is a drop in the energy supply, a defence reaction is activated and it will exploit every opportunity to build up its reserves.

Those who regularly go on reduced-calorie diets will know very well that the slightest lapse, at a weekend, for example, is all it needs to put back in one go the two or three kilos it has taken weeks of dieting to lose. This is one of the reasons why we advise you not to miss any meals. Depriving the body of food puts it into a state of alert which then makes it lay down reserves at the next meal. These reserves are what we want to avoid.

Interestingly enough, the habit of only feeding your dog once a day seems to be just as nonsensical as it is with a human. In most cases this explains over-weight in both humans and pets.

In addition, laboratory experiments with animals have shown that, with an identical daily food intake, animals which only had one meal a day put on weight, whereas no weight gain was seen among animals whose daily rations were divided between five or six meals. Less is, therefore, paradoxically, more. But don't forget that more is actually less!

The reduced calorie diet, which, as we've already shown, is illusory and ineffective, also has hidden dangers, because in the long term it consolidates overweight by increasing the number of fat cells.

If we look more closely at what happens with obesity – and here we're talk-ing about a weight that is more than 15 or 20 kilos above normal – we see in most cases that the excessive weight has been gained over several years as a result of a permanent reduced calorie way of eating.

In the following example you will see precisely how a stable starting weight of 90 kilos, with an intake of 3,000 calories, can suddenly turn into 120 kilos after several years, although the daily calorie intake was only 800. Let's look at this in more detail.

A reduced calorie diet goes through three stages:

- the weight-loss stage
- the stabilising stage
- the weight-gain stage

Also, unfortunately, with every new diet you try, the less weight you lose. Initially, you will almost regain your starting-weight, but then every new diet will lead to more weight gain.

For example, if you would really like to lose five kilos and do reach this goal, you will often find that you are 30 kilos overweight 15 years later, even though you have been eating low-calorie food all that time. That was not the point of the exercise.

Every day we hear doctors saying that patients have had no weight loss in spite of a strict diet (800 calories) and numerous sacrifices – most of them have even put on weight. There is an even greater problem as, during the diet, they suffer from a lack of essential nutrients:

- essential fatty acids
- mineral salts
- vitamins
- trace elements

and this results in severe fatigue and, particularly, in an increased susceptibility to illness, caused by a weakened immune system. Furthermore, patients suffered from attacks of depression, a voracious appetite and even anorexia. The only choice remaining to these women patients was to seek the help of a psychiatrist.

Moreover, such 'see-saw' diets encourage the development of heart disease and other circulatory problems even when there are no existing high levels of blood cholesterol (cholesterolemia) or diabetes present and the dieter is not a regular smoker.

There have been some impressive experiments to do with this. Professor Bronwell of the University of Pennsylvania has investigated this phenomenon in laboratory rats by alternately feeding them with low- and high-calorie food.

The animals experienced both weight loss and weight gain. There were differences in the duration of this, however. With the first diet the animals lost a certain amount of weight within three weeks and then put it back on again over the next 46 days. With the second diet the animals lost the same weight but the loss occurred over 56 days and they put back the weight within two weeks. After that it became harder and harder to achieve any weight loss and weight was gained much more quickly. This shows that the metabolism adjusts to the reduced calorie intake.

Certainly every reduction in calorie intake can lower the metabolic rate by more than 50%, yet every return to normal eating habits, even when it's only short-lived, inevitably leads to a drastic increase in weight.

Moreover, the bigger the difference between a diet and normal eating habits, the faster you put on weight again. The effect of these 'see-saw' diets, which make the weight fluctuate on the yo-yo principle, is very well known but, puzzlingly, specialists are very hesitant about bringing this into the open as if they had agreed on absolute silence. It is almost as if they are now afraid to admit that for 45 years they have been supporting a point of view which is completely mistaken.

Professor Apfelbaum made a welcome breakthrough, therefore, at the International Congress in Antwerp in September 1993, when he dared to ask the following question: 'Have we all been mistaken in our treatment of obesity?' To which he answered promptly: 'Yes!'

Strangely enough it is the people affected by obesity, those who have to suffer from it, who are still not prepared to accept the truth.

In the West, this 'reduced calorie intake phenomenon' has acquired a cultural significance which is firmly established in every sector of our society. How can we question a principle that is still on the curriculum of all medical faculties, which is propagated as the basis of dietetics teaching and which is used in all state institutions, hospitals, schools, and businesses? How can we question a principle that supports an important branch of industry in our Western world?

The food industry is booming; in some countries, France for example, it is the most important industry and one of the most successful.

When you visit a food fair you will find that the efforts of the industry in developing new products are concentrated on the reduced calorie way of eating. We see the same thing day in, day out, in advertisements that draw our attention to these reduced calorie products.

All market surveys are unambiguous: this is the way forward; this is the market of the future! The development of new products is geared to this. Even the hotel section has not escaped the 'virus' of reduced calorie food. In many hotels you can already find low-calorie dishes on the menu. Others have switched part of their hotel business over to reduced-calorie meals.

But it doesn't seem to be working. First and foremost we must admit to ourselves that the first step in the right direction is to recognise what we have been doing wrong. We need to query all those diets – the ones we've tried – or at least look at them from a different viewpoint. We also need to think of all the possible ways of reducing weight conventionally. So let us do that.

Why spend money for no reason?
Aids that are nothing of the kind

Those deceptive protein drinks

You probably know that the VLCD (Very Low Calories Diet) or diets based on protein drinks are included in the strictest reduced-calorie diets. These protein diets, which are intended for the most overweight cases, are unfortunately still prescribed by some doctors and used by many people without any medical supervision.

How protein drinks work

Instead of normal food 55g to 75g protein is taken in powder form (dissolved in liquids) or as a ready-prepared drink over a period of 20 to 30 days. These proteins supply about 500 calories a day (sometimes less!). As a supplement there are also vitamins and minerals and plenty of fluids (at least two litres a day).

Wasting of muscles is avoided through protein intake in these drinks; the lack of carbohydrates also decreases the blood-sugar level and the release of insulin. As a result, ketone bodies combine, which act within 48 hours to suppress the appetite and make the person concerned feel mildly euphoric.

The body is now forced to produce glucose from the fat reserves (this is called gluconeogenesis). Once the fat reserves are reduced (this is called lipolysis) weight will be lost.

This all sounds good. But where's the catch?

Scientific investigations into the individual parts of the body have revealed that some wasting of muscle does in fact occur in the first 19 days, and this only comes to a 'standstill' after the twentieth day.

Almost 25% of the weight loss that takes place can be attributed to this drop in muscle mass, though excessive weight does mean that there is a greater muscle mass. The considerable salt loss also promotes fluid excretion, which has an effect on the weight too. Care must be taken to avoid a drop in blood pressure. This hypotension (excessively low blood pressure) can be attributed to the missing carbohydrates, which bring about a decrease in the sodium and water balance.

After the diet has finished it is absolutely imperative to reintroduce carbo-hydrates gradually; if large quantities of them are absorbed, a high build-up of fluids will cause oedema.

VLCD has numerous side-effects:

- an increase in the level of uric acid: 10–20%
- hypotension: 8–10%
- hair loss: 9%
- constipation: 8–10%
- tiredness: 8%
- brittle nails: 8%
- dry skin: 8%
- sensitivity to cold: 8%
- muscle cramps: 7%
- depression: 5%
- headaches: 3%
- menstrual problems for women: 6%

The raised uric acid level (hyperuricaemia) lasts for roughly three weeks. To prevent the risks of attacks of gout or renal colic through the formation of urinary calculi (stones) it is extremely important to drink a lot of fluids. Con-stipation also frequently occurs; this can be helped by eating salad with a lemon juice dressing.

It is horrifying to know that these mixtures can be bought freely at pharma-cies, because they should normally only be prescribed for those people who are seriously overweight and who have had a thorough check of their heart and kidney function beforehand. There should be a gap of three months, by the way, before beginning another new diet.

It is also necessary to carry out such diets only under medical supervision, including a temporary in-patient visit and close monitoring of the heart.

Who can guarantee that those on the diet – intoxicated by their encouraging success – won't succumb to the temptation and continue with the treatment for longer than two months?

If this diet is only followed for a period of 8 to 10 days, all that will happen in the first week will be wasting of the muscles, fluid loss, and no decrease in fat, so you will basically get no slimmer!

In spite of making great sacrifices, there is no guarantee that you will lose any weight at all, as an investigation by Van Goal involving 400 people has shown. The success rates were only:

- 38% for six months
- 31% for one year
- 14% for two years

An investigation recently published by the University of Pennsylvania showed a success rate of only 2% after five years.

Professor Apfelbaum, a staunch advocate of this protein diet for more than 25 years, was brave enough to admit its ineffectiveness at the 'International Congress on the Phenomenon of Obesity' in Antwerp in September 1993, when he ended his speech with the words, 'In the long term, all those concerned had put back on the pounds they had lost'.

Worst of all, these treatments are widespread in spite of their risks (when they are used without medical checks), since they provide a lucrative business for the manufacturers and pharmacists. There is also a certain amount of commission when they are sold directly, after a doctor has prescribed them, so clearly we're not talking about small amounts of money here. Knowing this is part of our course in nutrition.

The main disadvantage of this slimming method, briefly, is that, for the dieters, it involves an artificial four-week interruption of their normal eating habits, which ignores the actual problem.

A long-term attempt to lose weight demands the co-operation of the patient and a diet method that is based on a fundamental, but not radical (!), change in our eating habits. Otherwise such a diet makes little sense.

Eat, yes, but in normal amounts. Only those things you buy at the grocer's, the market or the supermarket make sense; certainly don't shop in the pharmacy. You won't achieve a lasting, healthy or wholesome weight-loss from there.

What about these so-called meal replacements?

Nowadays we're inundated by slim people who tell us that they used to be plump but found the solution in some sort of drink that made them slim. It all sounds so easy. You take a glass, put in some powder and stir it and then. . . you lose weight.

If we look at the composition of such drinks, there are certain inconsistencies to be found; some have too little protein, others have too many 'bad' carbohydrates. All in all, fitness and slimming drinks like this make little sense long-term.

Let's have a closer look.

Those components of our human eating system which suppress hunger involve, on the one hand

- chewing and, secondly
- feeling full.

Chewing is not involved if you are just drinking, nor will you feel full. This is simply because fluids do not stay in the body long. A few hours later you will feel hungry again, so the risk is great that you will have a nibble of something between drinks. This also does not make you feel satisfied.

If we subsist on these 'meal replacements', especially at times when the risk of putting on fat is lowest – in other words in the morning and at lunchtimes – we will certainly eat more lavishly in the evening than we would normally. Why not? After all we've 'only' had fluids all day! Unfortunately, evening is the very time when our body tends to lay up fat reserves the most, especially when we've been deprived because we've missed a 'proper' meal. And deprived is the right word, because the body is not geared to this kind of unbalanced eating. Anyhow, that is the logic of a reduced calorie diet.

By using these meal replacements we unconsciously develop a kind of aversion to food. Subliminally we blame food for our weight problems.

In our minds we are convinced that food is our enemy. And it's before eating that we think we have to be careful, although in fact the opposite is the case!

We should get to like food instead of rejecting it wholesale. Of course, it is important to select the right things. But food can be our friend. Even in our everyday lives, we don't have to be good friends with all and sundry. And it's the same with food.

There's always some new miracle. . .
Aren't these miracle weight-loss cures just amazing

There's always some new miracle. . . And so we continue to dream of a wonder pill which will make our surplus fat melt like butter in the sun. What should such a wonder pill consist of? It must fulfil a couple of criteria to be both medically and ethically effective. It must:

- be proved to be effective by reliable, repeatable tests
- be well-tolerated (without undesirable side-effects)
- cause no symptoms of poisoning nor trigger any at any time

Unfortunately, that means we'll have to wait for this wonder pill for quite some time. Today there is not one single product that remotely meets these criteria. It's a real shame. And yet advertisements assure us again and again how easy it all is. . .

Let us have a closer look at the methods we are prescribed – or, unfortunately, still offered in the hope we'll lose weight.

Diuretic methods

If losing weight consists of losing a certain amount of fat, it is obvious that diuretics, which simply encourage water loss or, in other words, increase fluid excretion, do not fulfil this function in any way.

You also need to know that mineral salts (sodium, potassium) are excreted with the fluids as well, which in the long run does more harm than good. This leads to dry skin, tiredness, muscle cramps and attacks of dizziness with low blood pressure, which can cause fainting fits.

At the end of the course of treatment the body is likely to react like a dry sponge by absorbing water and salt as quickly as possible. This has the additional risk of leading to oedema, which can be hard to shift.

In this context beware of certain plant-based preparations, so-called 'dehydration methods', which consist of plants that to a greater or lesser degree encourage elimination of urine, thus giving the impression of a natural substance. Among these plants, for example, are hawkweed, horsetail, fennel, burdock, meadowsweet, artichokes, dandelion, ash and cherry stalks. They have perhaps only a slight diuretic effect, where less potassium is excreted, and yet they insist they only eliminate fluids...

Mineral water is often extolled as a slimming aid, but it only serves economic interests.

As has been mentioned already, it is certainly very important to drink a lot of fluid, but this only acts as a mild diuretic. Even when drinking leads to the excretion of the by-products of protein metabolism (urea, uric acid), this is far from being a reduction in fat!

Laxatives (aperients)

Some people think they lose weight when they gulp down laxatives! But taking laxatives can especially damage the large intestine or lead to a lack of potassium as a result of the diarrhoea that can accompany this 'purge'.

Thyroid extracts

An underactive thyroid is only responsible for obesity in exceptional cases. To prescribe thyroid extract for a patient whose thyroid is working perfectly will either have no effect or can actually be dangerous if this artificially makes the thyroid overactive.

These methods, which are more likely to lead to muscle wastage than to a decrease in fat, can also cause heart palpitations, for the heart is also a muscle, as we know (even if it's a very special one).

These thyroid extracts often disagree with the patient because of the side effects they cause (by destabilising the thyroid). Sometimes insomnia and panic attacks occur; the heart pounds or races and the patient trembles and becomes very agitated.

The worst complication, however, is when the heart suddenly decompensates (leading to a fall in blood pressure) if there is a previously existing coronary insufficiency (angina pectoris) that had perhaps not been discovered at an earlier examination.

Once again such 'poisons' are added to often complex preparations accompanied by complicated chemical descriptions or mysterious abbreviations. With plant-based preparations, for example, bladderwrack is used, which can have an effect on thyroid activity because of the iodine it contains.

Let us now move on to another favourite subject: appetite suppressants.

Appetite suppressants

These consist of appetite-suppressant amphetamines, which act as a strong stimulant on the personality. The agitation this produces can lead to sleep disturbances as well as reducing inhibitions.

Once the course of treatment is over depression or even suicide can occur but the worst thing is the resulting addiction. You can easily become dependent on appetite suppressants!

Overweight people, who often eat only small amounts of food, can usually avoid this, but, for those with eating problems (bulimia), taking amphetamines will make their condition worse.

In order to keep certain positive effects of amphetamines, efforts have been made to develop a medicine that has fewer risks. This has led to the dexfenfluramines, where the stimulating effect on the personality is no longer present. According to animal experiments they also no longer cause addiction.

They influence metabolic serotonin – a substance that affects the regulation of appetite – and bring about a feeling of repletion.

Dexfenfluramines have been shown to be effective for those who are addicted to sweet things, but this only applies to 15% of those who are overweight. It would therefore be wrong to use this as a valid treatment for everyone.

A series of experiments was carried out in which dexfenfluramines were used for a year to treat a group of more than 800 overweight women, of whom 86% were on average 40% heavier than their ideal theoretical weight.

A further control group of women were given placebos. Placebos are dummy medicines that have no effect. At the same time, those taking part were put on a medically supervised diet of less than 1,450 calories a day.

It turned out that the dexfenfluramine preparation disagreed with the patients. Almost 40% of the women had to abandon the treatment because of undesirable side effects. They suffered from fatigue, abdominal problems, headaches, sleep disturbances, diarrhoea, dry mouth, feelings of anxiety, depression, polyuria (chronic increase of urine excretion), giddy attacks, insomnia, sickness and vomiting.

After 11 months there was only a weight difference of about 2.7 kilos between the group that had been treated with the dexfenfluramines and the group who had been given placebos.

In a random survey, which took place two months after the end of the year-long treatment, it was found that the placebo group had gained a kilo a month and the dexfenfluramine group two kilos!

The doctors who had carried out the series of experiments concluded determinedly, and with an eye for profit, that the treatment should last for life, in order to maintain its relatively minor effectiveness – to the great delight of the manufacturer. . .

The results of this experiment throw up a few questions.

- Is it really necessary or, more especially, sensible to take two dexfenfluramine tablets daily for a whole year in order to lose 2.7 kilos more than if you took a placebo?

- Does this minimal success justify the horrendous cost of this treatment which private health insurance will not pay for?

- What effect would the medicine have had if it had been taken not in conjunction with a diet?
- How much of an effect in the end did the reduced calorie diet have combined with the psychological effect of the placebo?
- Are patients prepared to accept the risk of a slow weight-gain if they continue the one-year treatment, and the risk of a fast weight-gain if they stop taking dexfenfluramines?

Moreover, if more than a third of the 15% of overweight women in question have to break off their treatment early, in the final analysis only 10% of those taking part reap any benefits, by possibly losing three kilos more than they would with a conventional course of treatment.

Besides, no treatment for eating disorders could or should be confined to prescribing a medicine without including the necessary psychotherapy (or behavioural therapy) that should accompany a change in eating habits.

Even when lots of people would like a prescription of this 'wonder drug' because they want to lose weight as quickly as possible to be sure to be ready for summer on the beach, the doctor should still show caution. This is not about writing a hasty prescription in anticipation of a speedy success. This applies all the more to some medicines, apart from their poisonous content and undesirable side effects: after finishing the course of treatment female patients put back all the lost pounds again.

If this treatment is repeated regularly, the body activates its defence mechanism, which leads to a further increase in weight instead of the desired loss.

It must be emphasised again that a slimming method will only be successful if it is used long-term and if it is based on a change in existing eating habits.

Everyone wants a quick result

But quick results aren't possible where food is involved. After all we have taken years to reach our present weight, so it is only logical that we will need some time to reduce this weight.

We should beware of quick results just as we should beware of the countless slimming preparations that are wrongly marketed as natural products. Examples of these:

L-carnitine

L-carnitine is an enzyme that occurs in the body. Coming from the amino acids L-lysine and L-methionine, it is synthesised in the liver and kidneys with the help of iron and vitamins C and B_6. Nowadays it is rare to have an L-carnitine deficiency, since we get this enzyme from our normal food, for example, meat, chicken, rabbit, cow's milk and eggs. It is only among some female vegetarians, especially if they have an iron deficiency, where there can be too low a synthesis of L-carnitine.

Very rarely there is a congenital L-carnitine deficiency, but although those affected complain about muscle problems they are not overweight.

In advertisements L-carnitine is erroneously praised as a substance that promotes fat reduction. This must be corrected, for L-carnitine is required by the free fatty acids in the blood as 'fuel for energy' but in no way is it able to reduce fat reserves, which are stored as triglycerides. Only another enzyme, triglyceride lipase, which is activated by a low insulin level, makes a reduction of fat reserves and the removal of the resulting fatty acids, which pass into the bloodstream, possible.

Fortunately, the sales of numerous products containing L-carnitine have been banned.

Plants

Let us next look at preparations containing plants; plants which have a fat-reducing effect, teas which promote excretion of urine etc. They are all supremely suited giving the impression that weight can be lost without any great effort and that what you eat at the same time is unimportant!

Let's take bananas. Everyone has heard of the apparent fat-reducing effect of bananas. But the famous bromelin, which by the way is found in the stalk and not the fruit, in no way has this apparent capacity to make you slim. Contrary to what has been believed up to now, it does not even have a positive effect on insulin metabolism. And as for bean pods, they are no longer in vogue since they were discovered in the USA to be responsible for obstruction of the bowel.

Other plants, classified as harmless, have turned out to be poisonous – like germander for example, the sale of which is no longer permitted.

Some Chinese plants with fat-reducing properties (the more exotic the better) have caused severe hepatitis. The only substances that are acceptable at best are soluble fibres like Glucomannan, although in weak dosages this has absolutely no effect.

If a dose of four grams is taken daily, this helps to suppress the appetite. If it is taken with a lot of fluid half an hour before eating (it swells in the stomach) it will make you feel full in advance and it will decrease the release of insulin. However, it encourages agonising flatulence.

Whatever you take inevitably distracts you from your real goal, which is a lasting change in your eating habits. This change in the way you eat is the only possible means of stabilising your body weight in the long term.

What we eat, when we eat

What our food consists of

It is a matter of principle that we do not basically put on weight because we eat too much but because we are eating in the wrong way and do not choose the right foods.

The nutritional values in terms of energy, contained in food are not responsible for weight gain. Everything depends on what our food consists of. Food contains:

- carbohydrates
- fats
- proteins
- fibre
- vitamins
- mineral salts
- trace elements

In the final analysis it is pointless to eat less in order to get rid of excess pounds and reach your ideal weight if you go on eating the wrong food.

In order to change the way you eat, all you have to do is give up certain unhealthy foods and choose healthier foods instead. But to make the right choices it is vital to know your way round the food groups and to be able to recognise their distinctive features.

The great natural healer, Paracelsus, once said that everyone was their own doctor. And that's right. I alone really know what is good for my health and me.

But this knowledge doesn't just come out of the blue: we must work for it and, unfortunately, a little specialised knowledge is needed, too, so that we can understand the inner laws and mechanisms of food and its composition.

But, chin up, even if it does sometimes seem to be very theoretical, you can catch a glimpse of your reward in the distance:

- a more detailed and better understanding of your own nutrition and, therefore,
- a healthier and more active life!

What are foods?

What are foods actually? Foods are edible substances that contain a certain number of nutrients, such as:

- proteins
- lipids
- carbohydrates

They also contain:

- water
- indigestible substances such as
  - fibre
  - micronutrients:
    vitamins
    mineral salts
    trace elements

Foods can also be divided into two basic groups:

- nutrients which provide energy
- those which do not

These energy-providing nutrients act as a source of energy and as raw material for numerous physical processes that occur during the formation and reformation of living tissues. Included here are proteins, lipids and carbohydrates.

Those nutrients that do not provide energy are needed for the absorption and metabolism of energy-providing nutrients. Some trigger or act as catalysts for chemical reactions in the body. We can differentiate between fibre (roughage), water, mineral salts, trace elements and vitamins.

Armed with this knowledge, we can now have a look at our list of nutrients. Let's turn first to proteins.

Proteins (or albumens)

Proteins are the organic components of living cells and tissues. They form the structure of the muscles, liver, brain, bones etc. They consist of simpler molecules, called 'amino acids', some of which are produced by the body. However, the amino acids most needed by the body are obtained through food, where protein has two sources:

- animal or
- vegetable

Animal protein can be found in:

- meat
- fish
- cheese
- eggs
- sausage
- shellfish
- mussels
- offal
- milk products

Vegetable protein can be found in:

- soya
- almonds
- hazelnuts
- whole-wheat
- chocolate
- algae
- cereals
- wholegrain products
- some pulses (beans, lentils)

It is therefore important to ensure an adequate intake of proteins, as they are necessary:

- for the formation of cell structures, the production of certain hormones and neurotransmitters (neurotransmitters are chemical substances, released from stimulated nerve endings which have a corresponding biological effect)
- for the creation of nucleic acids (necessary for reproduction)
- as a possible source of energy after conversion to glucose (Krebs cycle)

In passing: no other food is such an ample and balanced source of amino acids as the egg! When you learn that the lack of one vital amino acid can disrupt the absorption of others, you will understand better why we should eat both animal and vegetable foods.

An exclusively vegetarian diet can lead to an imbalance in the body. This, however, is not the case when a meatless diet is supplemented by egg and milk products. In contrast to this, a protein intake that is obtained exclusively through meat will lead to a deficiency in sulphur-containing amino acids, which can disrupt the absorption of other amino acids.

For a balanced diet an adult should have 1g of protein per kilo of body weight daily; the daily minimum should be 60g for women and 70g for men. Protein should also make up 15% of our daily food intake. Children need at least 60g of protein a day and young people need 90g.

The intake of protein can also be higher than this (1.2 to 1.5g of protein per kilo of body weight per day), provided you drink enough to eliminate the metabolic waste products of protein (uric acid, urea). An increase in protein intake during the weight-loss stage can be a very effective help. The absorption of albumen in the metabolism uses up more energy than when other nutrients are absorbed and results more quickly in a satisfying feeling of fullness. As a result of regulating mechanisms, according to Professor D. Tome, adults can have a varying intake of protein, between 0.6 and 2.0g per kilogram of body weight, per day, without this having any great repercussions for their health. Table 1 shows us clearly which foods contain protein.

Table: Foods Containing Protein		
	Animal Proteins	**Vegetable Proteins**
Average Concentrations	beef veal lamb pork poultry sausage fish mature cheese	soya beans wholegrains algae roast peanuts lentils white beans almonds
High Concentration	eggs milk curd cheese	oats 100% wholegrain bread chocolate (more than 70% cocoa wholegrain rye pasta whole rice walnuts lentils

Ideally we should eat as much vegetable protein as animal protein. However, this is not always easy.

An inadequate intake of protein from food can have serious consequences for the body:

- muscle wastage
- weakening of our defence system
- wrinkled skin
- bad scarring
- organ damage

When, on the other hand, too much protein is obtained from food, protein waste products remain in the body, including uric acid, which can lead to gout. We need, therefore, to drink a lot of fluids in order to flush out these waste products.

Proteins are necessary for our health. Even an excess of protein usually presents no problem, unless kidney function is already damaged. Also, proteins are generally linked in food with fats (lipids), which are usually saturated and which should only be eaten in very small quantities.

Carbohydrates

Let us look at carbohydrates. Carbohydrates are molecules that consist of carbon, hydrogen and oxygen. They are converted by the metabolism into glucose, an important source of energy for the body and one that is quickly mobilised for use.

Carbohydrates can be divided into various types, depending on the chemical complexity of their molecules. Let us get to know them better.

⇨ **Carbohydrates with one molecule** (monosaccharides)

- glucose (from the Greek *glukus* 'sweet'), which is found in small quantities in honey and fruit
- fructose, which is mainly found in fruit
- galactose, which is contained in milk

⇨ **Carbohydrates with two molecules** (disaccharides)

- sucrose, which is nothing more than white sugar (granulated sugar, sugar cubes); it is produced from sugar beet or sugar cane (glucose + fructose)
- lactose (glucose + galactose), which is found in mammal's milk

41

- maltose (glucose + glucose) which is made from malts, i.e. from beer and maize
⇨ **Carbohydrates with several molecules** (polysaccharides)
  - glycogen, found in animal liver
  - starch which is combined from numerous glucose molecules and is found in the following foods:
    ○ cereals: wheat, maize, rice, rye, barley, oats
    ○ tubers: potatoes, yams
    ○ root vegetables: swedes, turnips
    ○ grains and pulses: chick peas, dried beans, soya beans

Cellulose, hemicellulose, pectin, vegetable flours and thickeners can also be included, as we are dealing here with carbohydrates that cannot be absorbed during digestion. They therefore provide no energy for the body. They are better classified with fibre.

For a long time, carbohydrates were divided into two different categories, according to the supposed speed by which they were assimilated by the body:

- fast sugars on one hand and
- slow sugars on the other

Under the heading 'fast sugars' were found the simple and double sugars like glucose and sucrose, which occur in refined sugars (cane or beet sugar) and in honey and fruit. They are speedily converted in the digestive tract and quickly absorbed in the small intestine, very soon after they have been eaten.

On the other hand, there were those carbohydrates that were assigned to the 'slow sugars' category, as it was assumed that their complex molecule was chemically converted into simple sugar (glucose) during the course of digestion. This particularly applies to the starch of starch-containing foods; glucose from these is released more slowly and in stages. This categorisation is totally out-dated nowadays, because it is based on a false assumption.

Most recent investigations show that the complexity of the carbohydrate molecule has no effect on the speed with which the glucose is released and assimilated by the body.

In the meantime, it has also been found that the blood-sugar peak of all carbohydrates (in other words, their maximum absorption) is reached equally fast for all of them, i.e. about 30 minutes after food has been eaten on an empty stomach.

Figure 2 Rate of absorption of carbohydrates

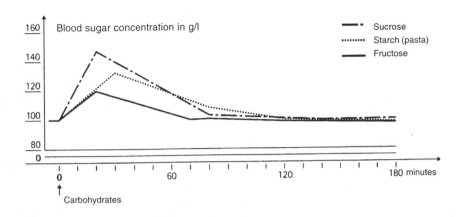

Figure 2 shows very nicely how quickly carbohydrates are used, or absorbed, by the body. However, instead of investigating the speed of assimilation, we should be looking at the effect carbohydrates have in raising blood-sugar levels, i.e. the quantity of glucose produced.

Nowadays all scientists agree that carbohydrates should be classified according to their hyperglycaemic (increase in blood sugar) effect, which is determined by the glycaemic index.

This concept of 'glycaemic index' is so central to the Montignac Method and will become so essential to it that we must look at it in detail.

Sweet blood!
What is glycaemia?

Glucose is an important 'fuel' for the body. It is imperative for the functioning of the brain.

Glucose is produced in two ways:

- it is synthesised by the body when the fat reserves are broken down or
- it is formed in the metabolism of carbohydrates

Glucose is always transported via the blood (stored, or not, as glycogen). It is therefore always present in the blood. Glycaemia shows the amount of glucose contained in the blood.

Thus, 'glycaemia' means the glucose content of the blood, which, on an empty stomach, is 'normally' one gram of glucose per litre of blood. If the glycaemia falls below this level, it is returned to normal by the secretion of the pancreatic hormone glucagon. When you eat carbohydrates, the corresponding absorption of glucose leads to a rise in glycaemia.

After carbohydrates have been eaten on an empty stomach, the change in blood-sugar levels is easily seen, as Figure 3 shows.

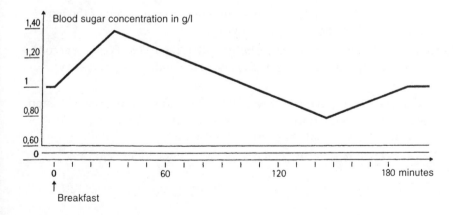

Figure 3

At first the blood-sugar level rises more or less depending on the type of carbohydrate until its maximum level, the so-called glycaemic or blood-sugar high, is reached. The pancreas, which plays an important part in the regulating of the metabolic processes, then secrates the hormone insulin, so that excessive glucose passes from the blood into the cells (liver, muscles), where it can be used if needed. Thus insulin lowers the blood-sugar level, which eventually returns to normal.

The glycaemic index

The glycaemic potential of each carbohydrate is defined by its glycaemic amplitude and measured on the glycaemic index developed by Prof. Crapo in the USA in 1976.

The glycaemic index corresponds to the area of the triangle of the hyperglycaemic or blood-sugar graph, which is triggered by the carbohydrate that has been eaten.

Glucose arbitrarily keeps the index 100, which represents the area of the triangle of the corresponding hyperglycaemic curve.

The following formula is used to calculate the glycaemic index of the remaining carbohydrates:

$$\frac{\text{Area of triangle of tested carbohydrate x 100}}{\text{Area of triangle of glucose}}$$

The glycaemic index is all the higher depending on the extent of the hyperglycaemia caused by the tested carbohydrate.

Today most scientists agree that carbohydrates should be classified according to their ability – determined by the glycaemic index – to increase blood-sugar levels.

The glycaemic index provides us with the explanation for the phenomenon of obesity and for numerous other problems such as tiredness and lack of energy, which many people have to contend with.

Figures 4 and 5 illustrate a high and a low glycaemic index.

Figure 4 High glycaemic index

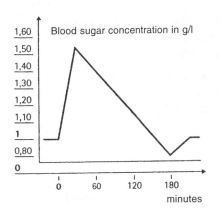

Figure 5 Low glycaemic index

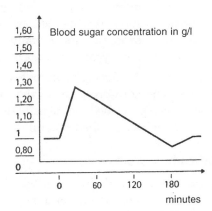

It has been discovered that the glycaemic index of carbohydrates rises after industrial processing as well as certain other methods of preparation (corn-flakes, 85; maize, 70: instant potato, 95; boiled potatoes, 70).

It was also established that the glycaemic index of food containing carbohydrate depends not only on the composition of the starch (proportion of amylose/amylopectin) but also on the quantity of proteins and fibre contained, and the type of fibre (very white hamburger baps, 95; white bread, baguette, 70; wholemeal bread, 50; wholegrain bread, 40; white rice, 70; brown rice, 50).

For simplicity's sake we can divide carbohydrates into two categories:

- 'good' carbohydrates with a low glycaemic index
- 'bad' carbohydrates with a high glycaemic index

With this distinction in mind we will find the real reasons for excess weight in the following chapters.

Let us now look at these categories we have just established of 'good' and 'bad' carbohydrates.

'Bad' carbohydrates

In this category we can include all carbohydrates whose assimilation leads to a sharp rise of glucose in the blood and so to hyperglycaemia.

This applies to all forms of white sugar (pure or in combination with other foods such as in biscuits etc.) and also for all carbohydrates from white flour (white bread, pasta) and white rice, as well as foods using potatoes and corn that have been processed industrially. This applies particularly to carbohydrates where the glycaemic index is above 50.

This category of 'bad' carbohydrates also includes certain popular foods such as potatoes and corn products, as their glycaemic index is far higher when they have been processed industrially (potato starch, crisps, cornflakes, popcorn. . .) or cooked (mashed potato).

'Good' carbohydrates

In contrast to 'bad' carbohydrates, 'good' carbohydrates are only assimilated by the body to a small degree and they therefore only lead to a slight increase of glucose in the blood (glycaemia).

This is the case with wholegrains (high-fibre flour), wholegrain rice, certain pulses like lentils and dried beans, and above all with most fruits and all vegetables, which also come under the heading of high-fibre foods (leeks, cabbage, broccoli, cauliflower, salads, green beans) and which all contain a certain amount of carbohydrate.

Hyperglycaemia and insulin

To complete the picture: when the absorption of a carbohydrate has reached its highest point (blood-sugar peak), the pancreas separates the insulin hormone, which has the task of driving the glucose out of the blood so that the blood-sugar level drops again (as has already been described). The quantity of insulin produced inevitably relates to the height of the blood-sugar level; in most cases hyperglycaemia leads to 'hyperinsulinism'.

Later we will return in greater detail to this concept, which is very important for understanding exactly the majority of metabolic processes and their effects – especially on weight gain.

Table 2 Glycaemic index table

Carbohydrates with a high glycaemic index		Carbohydrates with a low glycaemic index	
maltose (beer)	110	wholegrain or bran bread	50
glucose	100	whole rice	50
sauté potatoes	95	basmati rice (long grain)	50
chips	95	tinned peas	50
ground rice	95	sweet potatoes	50
modified starch	95	wholegrain pasta (whole wheat)	50
instant mashed potato mix	90	spaghetti (al dente)	45
crisps	90	fresh peas	40
honey	85	wholegrain cereals without sugar	40
very white bread (burger bun)	85	oats	40
cooked carrots	85	kidney beans	40
cornflakes, popcorn	85	fresh fruit juice without sugar	40
easy-cook long grain rice	85	pumpernickel (dark rye bread)	40
rice pudding	85	100% wholegrain bread	40
puffed rice	85	ice-cream	40
cooked broad beans	80	wholegrain pasta (al dente)	40
water melon	75	figs, dried apricots	35
pumpkin	75	Indian corn	35
sugar (sucrose)	70	wild rice	35
white bread (baguette)	70	quinoa	35
refined cereals with sugar	70	raw carrots	30
chocolate bars	70	milk products	30
(peeled) boiled potatoes	70	dried beans	30
coca cola, lemonade	70	brown/yellow lentils	30
biscuits	70	chick peas	30
corn, maize	70	other fresh fruits	30
white rice	70	green beans	30
pasta, ravioli	70	fine Chinese noodles (soya)	30
raisins	65	sugar-free jam	22
bread (mixed flours)	65	green lentils	22
(unpeeled) boiled potatoes	65	dried peas	22
turnips	65	dark chocolate (>70% cocoa)	22
jam with sugar	65	fructose	20
semolina	60	soya, peanuts	15
long grain rice	60	fresh apricots	15
banana, melon	60	green vegetables, tomatoes	< 15
white spaghetti, cooked till soft	55	aubergines, courgettes	
cakes (Madeira sponge)	55	garlic, onions	

The other things we eat
Don't be afraid of fatty fats!

Lipids or fats

In the Western world, for some time now, fats have triggered a real psychosis; in the USA the behaviour of the population verges on paranoia.

Once, for hundreds of years, fat was the most highly coveted and the most highly regarded food; today it is the target for accusations and calls for its rejection.

Traditional dietetics teaching blames fats first and foremost for obesity, because they contain a large number of calories. It was also able to believe that fat triggers most coronary and circulatory illnesses through cholesterol. Fat is even accused today of playing an important role in the formation of certain types of cancer.

Lipids are complex molecules that, above all, contain fatty acids. Two large groups of lipids can be distinguished according to their origin:

⇨ **lipids of animal origin** are contained in:

- meat
- fish
- butter
- eggs
- cheese
- milk products etc.

⇨ **lipids of vegetable origin** are contained in:

- groundnut oil
- olive oil
- walnut oil
- sunflower oil
- margarine etc.

Lipids can also be placed in three categories depending on the type of fatty acids:

⇨ **saturated fatty acids,** contained in
- meat
- sausages, salami, ham. . .
- eggs
- wholemilk products (milk, butter, cream, cheese)

⇨ **monounsaturated fatty acids,** contained especially in :
- olive oil
- goose fat
- duck fat
- pâté de foie gras

⇨ **polyunsaturated vegetable fatty acids,** contained in
- oil produced from seeds (especially sunflower oil)
- oil-bearing crops
- Polyunsaturated fatty acids are industrially hardened in the manufacture of margarine by hydrogenation.

⇨ **polyunsaturated animal fatty acids,** contained especially in
- fish
- shellfish

Lipids are *indispensable food components, they*:
- provide energy which can be stored in the form of fatty acids and which are readily available to supply the body with energy
- are the starting point for the formation of membranes and cells
- are components of tissues and, especially, the nervous system
- enable the formation of hormones and prostaglandin
- provide the basic material for the formation of gall salts
- are the carriers of the fat-soluble vitamins A, D, E and K
- are the only source of the so-called essential fatty acids linoleic acid and a-linolenic acid
- help to prevent cardiovascular diseases (some fatty acids)

Later on we will see that we have to distinguish between 'good' and 'bad' fats as well. Fatty foods also contain numerous vitamins (A, D, E, K) as well as essential fatty acids (linoleic acid and linolenic acid) and facilitate the manufacture of various hormones.

We often use too much fat in cooking, for example, when we fry and deep-fat fry, or when we make unnecessary sauces, although dishes that are just as delicious can be prepared with less fat.

Some lipids lead to too high a blood-cholesterol level. There really is 'good' and 'bad' cholesterol. The point for us is to keep our overall cholesterol at a normal level by trying to create optimal conditions, so that the concentration of 'good' cholesterol (HDL cholesterol) stays as high as possible while we keep that of 'bad' cholesterol (LDL) as low as possible. We need to know that not all fats lead to a rise in 'bad' cholesterol. There are even fats which cause a noticeable drop.

It is useful to *divide fats into three categories, according to their characteristics:*

⇨ **Fats which may raise the cholesterol level.** These are saturated fats, found in:

- meat
- sausages
- butter
- cheese
- lard
- wholemilk products
- palm oil

Too great an intake of saturated fatty acids can lead to an increase in cholesterol levels in the blood, which can encourage cardiovascular diseases. Numerous investigations also expressed the opinion that an excessive consumption of saturated fatty acids can become a risk factor in the development of certain types of cancers.

⇨ **Fats which have little impact on cholesterol levels.** They are found in:

- poultry (skin removed)
- seafood
- eggs

⇨ **Fats which lower the cholesterol level.** These are:

- plant oils
  olive oil, rapeseed oil, sunflower oil, corn oil etc.

Fish oils have little real influence on cholesterol metabolism, but they prevent cardiovascular diseases, since they lower the level of triglycerides and prevent thrombosis. You should, therefore, eat oily fish (salmon, tuna, mackerel, herring and sardines).

The method suggested in this book for losing weight is based principally on making the right choice between 'good' and 'bad' carbohydrates. In the same way you have to choose between 'good' and 'bad' fats if your cholesterol level tends to be high, in order to protect yourself permanently against this particular risk and against cardiovascular diseases in general.

Lipids and obesity

Fats are the greatest providers of energy, which is why reduced-calorie diets regard them as the greatest enemy.

But as we shall show later, it is not so much the amount of energy that we have to be scare of when eating, as bad eating habits, which destabilise our metabolism and encourage the laying down of fat reserves. It is, therefore, hyperglycaemia, via hyperinsulinism, that contributes to the storage of excessive amounts of fat (lipogenesis).

Lipids and cholesterol

There really is an interaction between an excessive consumption of fat and the cholesterol level in the blood (responsible for cardiovascular diseases). However, we need to make a distinction here, for the overall cholesterol in the blood is divided into two types of cholesterol: 'good' and 'bad' cholesterol.

An ideal cholesterol level is two grams per litre at most, whereas the concentration of 'good' cholesterol should be as high as possible.

We distinguish between:

- **monounsaturated fatty acids,** especially those from olive oil, which are capable of lowering overall cholesterol and increasing 'good' cholesterol. They have the advantage of being chemically stable.

- **polyunsaturated fatty acids** which are found especially in sunflower oil, corn and rapeseed oil and which can lower the overall level of cholesterol. They are rich in essential fatty acids, but have the disadvantage that they are easily oxidised. Once oxidised, they are just as harmful for the vascular walls as saturated fatty acids.

The same occurs with some vegetable fats, which are chemically changed when hardened (in the manufacture of margarine) and therefore seem to change their characteristics.

Essential fatty acids

Linoleic acid and a-linolenic acid (previously called 'Vitamin F') deserve special attention here, because they are absolutely vital for nutrition.

In the last few years, the fundamental significance of these fatty acids in the formation of brain cell membranes and the development of the nervous system has been clearly established. A lack of these fatty acids must therefore lead to damage to intellectual development, especially if this lack occurs in early childhood.

It has also been shown that a deficiency of these fatty acids can play a decisive role in the development of the most serious metabolic illnesses which afflict industrialised countries, and which particularly include diseases of the immune system.

It is probably our bad modern eating habits that are responsible for this deficiency; habits like the consumption of products of a dubious nature, especially when they are highly refined. Linoleic acid, which is found in sunflower oil, corn oil and grapeseed oil, lowers the risk of coronary and circulatory diseases.

A lack of this fatty acid leads to growth problems and changes to the cells in the skin, mucous membranes, endocrine glands and sexual organs. The recommended intake is 10g per day, which can be obtained, for example, from 20g of sunflower oil, corn oil or soya oil.

A-linolenic acid, which is found in large quantities in rapeseed oil, walnut oil and wheatgerm oil, is especially important for the chemical processes in the nervous system. A lack of this acid can lead to disturbances in learning ability, abnormalities in nerve conductivity, a heightened risk of thrombosis and a reduced tolerance to alcohol. The recommended intake is 2g per day, which can be obtained, for example, from 25g of rapeseed oil.

The consumption of a single oil is not enough to maintain a balanced amount of fatty acids, linoleic acid and a-linolenic acid. You should therefore mix two or three types of oil (or vary them) for a salad dressing. You should use one of the following:

- olive oil + Isio 4 (a mixture of soya oil, grapeseed oil and predominantly two types of sunflower oil; produced in France by Lesieur)
- olive oil + sunflower oil + rapeseed oil

Daily fat intake

Daily total fat intake should not represent more than 30% of our total food intake. Ideally, fat intake should be divided between 25% saturated fats (meat, sausage, butter, whole milk products), 50% monounsaturated fatty acids (goose fat, olive oil) and 25% polyunsaturated fatty acids (fish, sunflower oil, rape-seed oil, corn oil, etc.).

Here we have shown in some detail how difficult it is to achieve balance in food and how easily prejudices and wrong ideas can even lead to health problems.

The fact that certain nutriments are not sources of energy in no way lessens their usefulness in food. The opposite is the case. But the fact that they provide no energy has caused many of our contemporaries to neglect them, although they play a vital role in nutrition.

Our ancestors ate fibre without knowing it. We only discovered it a short while ago and, in doing so, realised we eat too little of it.

Dietary fibre

Fibre is predominantly contained in carbohydrates with a low glycaemic index, in other words, in vegetables, pulses, fruit, high-fibre cereals and in so-called wholefoods. It supplies no additional calories, but plays an extremely important role in digestion. It reduces the absorption of carbohydrates and, therefore, glycaemia.

There are two types of fibre:

- **insolublefibre** (cellulose, hemicellulose) shortens transit time (the time taken between eating and excretion) and prevents constipation
- **soluble fibre** (vegetable flours and thickeners, pectins) reduces the absorption of lipids in the intestines and thus prevents arteriosclerosis

Insoluble fibre sucks up water like a sponge and thus brings about a faster emptying of the stomach and an increase in the volume and water content of the contents of the bowel, which improves excretion.

Its basic significance lies, therefore, in the avoidance of constipation (together with an ample intake of fluids). It also contributes to a slight reduction of the cholesterol level in the blood and is particularly effective in preventing the formation of gallstones. Finally, it can have a preventive effect against cancers of the large intestine and the rectum, which still cause many deaths every year!

In the past phytic acid, which is contained in cereal grains, was accused of inhibiting the absorption of calcium. As a consequence, it was said that '100% wholegrain bread causes a calcium deficiency'. More recent research, however, has shown that this is not the case, especially when bread is made with a raising agent and in the traditional way (without kneading to speed up the process).

Fibre also does not affect the absorption of vitamins and trace elements, especially as high-fibre foods (fruit, pulses, vegetables) often contain large amounts of these micronutrients, which are imperative for our bodies to function without problems.

Soluble fibre absorbs very large quantities of water, which results in the formation of a very thick pulp. With its large volume, this pulp fills the stomach to a large extent, which quickly produces a feeling of repletion. Consequently, the feeling of hunger disappears more quickly without any calories being added. This pulp regulates the absorption of carbohydrates and fats. There is, therefore, not such a pronounced rise in the blood-sugar level after the consumption of food rich in soluble fibre, although the same quantity of carbohydrates is digested. Less insulin is also released. This hormone encourages the formation of fat reserves, i.e. weight gain. All in all, soluble fibre can achieve weight loss when substantial amounts of food are eaten.

This process can also bring about an improvement in diabetes, since a lowering of the blood-sugar level occurs. Diabetics should therefore preferably eat foods containing carbohydrates that are rich in fibre (fruit, haricot beans and especially lentils) and which have a low glycaemic index.

Fibre lowers the cholesterol level in the blood and so protects against cardiovascular diseases. This is all the more so as certain high-fibre foods (vegetables, raw fruits and oil-bearing crops) contain antioxidants (vitamins C and E, beta carotene) which, in addition, protect the vascular walls. This positive effect on the blood fats also applies to triglycerides. Unfortunately, far too little fibre is eaten in all industrialised countries, especially the USA. Thirty grams would just about be adequate, but it should be 40g per day.

High-fibre foods contain many vitamins, trace elements and mineral salts and a lack of these can lead to serious deficiency symptoms. One advantage of fibre is that it can limit the toxic effects of some chemical substances, such as dyes and additives. Medical specialists believe that some types of fibre also protect against bowel and rectal cancers. The increased standard of living in the Western world over the last few decades has led to a sharp drop in the consumption of fibre. In 1925 the consumption per head of pulses (which are particularly high in fibre) in France was 7.3kg. Today it is 1.3kg, 5.6 times lower.

Pasta has long been the basis of Italian cooking. Thirty years ago most meals consisted of vegetables (rich in fibre) and wholegrain foods that contained wheat fibre. As living standards rose, pulses and vegetables were mostly replaced by meat. Pasta was manufactured with low-fibre white flour, from which fibre had been removed. As a result, health authorities in Italy have recorded an alarming increase in obesity and bowel cancer.

Table 3 Sources of fibre (content in 100g food)

Cereal products		Pulses		Dried fruit with oils	
bran	40g	dried beans	25g	dried coconut	25g
wholegrain bread	13g	dried peas	23g	dried figs	18g
wholegrain flour	9g	lentils	12g	almonds	14g
white bread	2.5g	peanuts	8g	dates	9g
whole rice	1g	chick peas	2g	raisins	7g
Green vegetables		**Green vegetables**		**Fresh fruits**	
parsley	19g	cabbage	4g	raspberries	8g
cooked peas	12g	radishes	3g	pear (unpeeled)	3g
cooked spinach	7g	mushrooms	2.5g	apple (unpeeled)	3g
lamb's lettuce	5g	carrots	2g	strawberries	2g
artichokes	4g	lettuce	2g	peach	2g
leeks	4g				

It has been shown that fibre indirectly has a positive influence on obesity. Its presence in food lowers glycaemia and insulinaemia, in other words, the insulin content in the blood, which is responsible for the formation of fat reserves. Figures 6 and 7 show that insulinaemia is reduced when carbohydrates with a high glycaemic index are eaten together with fibre.

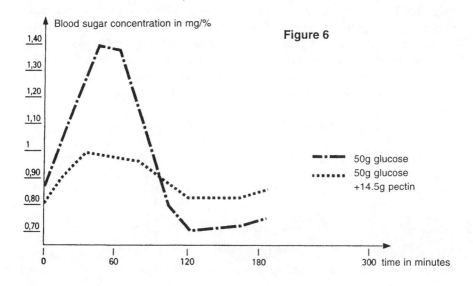

Figure 6

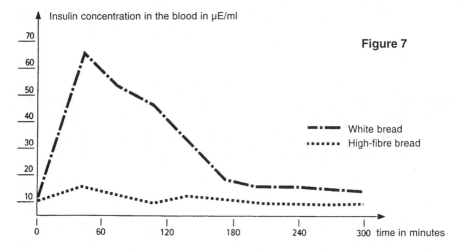

Figure 7

Water

The amount of water in a healthy adult's body makes up 45 to 65% of their weight. Human beings can manage for weeks without food but only a few days without water.

They can lose their glycogen and fat reserves and half of their protein and not be exposed to a serious risk but a 10% water loss would cause considerable exhaustion.

Everyone knows that water loss caused by urination, breathing, perspiration and evacuation of the bowels must be replaced. This excretion of water amounts to between two and two and a half litres per day.

This replacement occurs through:

- drinks: 1.5 litres per day (water, skimmed milk, fruit juice, tea, soup. . .)
- fluid contained in solid food (for example, bread consists of 35% water)
- metabolic fluid, i.e. fluid which occurs as a result of the various chemical processes in the body

A sufficient water intake is indicated by the pale colour of urine. If the urine is dark, however, this is a clear sign that too little has been drunk.

Mineral salts and trace elements

Mineral salts are vital substances. They are involved in the metabolism and in the electro-chemical processes of the nerve and muscle system as well as the formation of bones, teeth and other tissues. Some minerals also function as catalysts in numerous chemical reactions in the body.

Minerals are divided into two groups:

- minerals which are needed by the body in relatively large quantities: macrominerals
- minerals present in tiny quantities: trace elements

These substances act as catalysts in chemical reactions in the body. They are carriers, so to speak, which assist the enzymes in their work. If they are missing, the chemical reactions cannot take place. These substances are, therefore, absolutely essential, even though they only have to be present in extremely small amounts.

Some trace elements have been known about for a long time – iron, for example. Its significance for health was recognised as far back as the world of the ancients, although no one knew how this effect came about.

Most trace elements, however, have only been discovered recently in tests carried out into 'illnesses caused by civilisation' (such as lack of energy or tiredness).

Mineral salts	Trace elements
sodium	iron
potassium	iodine
calcium	zinc
phosphorus	copper
magnesium	manganese
	fluoride
	chromium
	selenium
	cobalt
	molybdenum

Table 4

Trace elements are metals or metalloids, which are present in the body in very small quantities. Nowadays there are problems with trace elements regarding quantity and quality. As a result of intensive industrial cultivation in the form of a massive use of artificial fertilisers and phosphates and a failure to include natural fertilisers in the biological cycle the soil is low in trace elements. This is particularly true of manganese.

The plants growing in this exhausted soil contain too few trace elements as well. Even the animal world is affected: in some cases an additional intake of zinc is needed to ensure reproduction, for example, in cattle; without zinc no procreation can take place. Since our foods contain ever fewer trace elements, a deficiency occurs in our body. A large number of specialists believe that our modern illnesses can be put down to this deficiency.

Two possibilities present themselves: we either go back to traditional methods, as has been successfully done with organic methods of cultivation, or we supplement our food with food additives until a method of cultivation can be used that relates better to our natural needs.

Vitamins

Over the centuries, in exceptional situations (sieges, famines, sea voyages), certain illnesses were seen which were obviously connected with bad nutrition. This applied, for example, to bleeding of the gums (a sign of scurvy), abnormalities of the bone (a sign of rickets), paralysis and oedema (a sign of beriberi) or injuries to the skin (a sign of pellagra).

Only around the turn of the last century could it be proved that this imbalance could be ascribed to the lack of essential substances, described as vitamins, in the diet.

With the change of eating habits in the last few decades, the generally widespread consumption of refined products (white sugar, white flour, white rice) and the development of high-yield plants, which are industrially processed, more and more frequent cases of vitamin deficiency have been found. Vitamins could almost be defined as organic compounds that are essential in small amounts to maintain life, promote growth and ensure the procreation of humans and the majority of animals.

They occur in several foods. Lean meat, for example, and offal especially (liver and kidneys), which contain large amounts, are a good source of vitamins. Seeds and grains such as pulses, walnuts, hazelnuts or cereals are also very rich in vitamins, but root vegetables and tubers (potatoes) are less so. The vitamin content in fruit and fresh vegetables varies according to the composition of the soil, the time of year and the way they are stored and prepared.

Although it is interesting to speak of vitamins as a whole, they do form a heterogeneous group because of their structure and their effect. Therefore it is useful to look at them separately. There is an obvious division into two groups: fat-soluble vitamins and water-soluble vitamins.

⇨ **Fat-soluble vitamins**

There are four fat-soluble vitamins: A, D, E and K. In general they are contained in fatty foods, in butter, cream, vegetable oils, fats and certain types of vegetables. They have the following characteristics in common:

- they are heat-resistant
- they are stored in the body, especially in the liver; in consequence, deficiencies are slow to occur
- they can be toxic if taken in large quantities (especially vitamins A and D)

⇨ **Water-soluble vitamins**

As these vitamins are water-soluble they can be excreted via the urinary tract in the event of a surplus. Although they have differing characteristics, they are closely connected with each other through the various cell reactions in which they are involved. The following are among the most important water-soluble vitamins:

- vitamin C: ascorbic acid
- vitamin B_1: thiamine
- vitamin B_2: riboflavin

- vitamin PP: niacin
- vitamin B_5: pantothenic acid
- vitamin B_6: pyridoxine
- vitamin B_8: biotin
- vitamin B_9: folic acid
- vitamin B_{12}: cyanacobalamin

Like the trace elements, vitamins also function as catalysts as part of numerous biochemical reactions. Nowadays the effects of a vitamin deficiency are fairly well known; in most cases the symptoms are obvious.

On the other hand, less well known are the details of their interrelationship and the precise effects of a deficiency.

However, the knowledge that we do possess is very considerable. Because of this knowledge, which becomes more extensive from day to day, it is impossible not to feel affected. For this reason we should ask the right questions and make sure that they are answered.

The following chapters will show that overweight is caused more by a destabilised metabolism than by too large a quantity of food, which is what we hear far too often.

We will particularly see that a drastic reduction in our daily food intake, as is the intention of reduced calorie diets, can only lead to a worsening of the mineral and vitamin deficiency already evident in our food. Astonishingly, it is these very diets, reduced in calories, which trigger one deficiency after the other and so lead to the emergence of obesity.

The following chapters will be concerned with developing an awareness of these connections and with turning this knowledge we have acquired into action, in order to limit the negative effects as much as possible.

With what you now know about the composition of food you will be able to understand why you put on weight and how you can eat and, at the same time, slim the right way, permanently.

May we have more?
Why <u>do</u> we put on weight?

Anyone who has tried to eat less in order to lose weight will have discovered that this target cannot be achieved permanently. Instead of losing the excess pounds forever, a few months later the scales will often show that you weigh more than before.

We have been able to show that it is not the excessive energy intake through our food which is responsible for the formation of fat reserves, but the composition of the food eaten, i.e. the composition of its nutrients.

Conventional dietetics, which is based on reduced calorie intake, assumes that the reason we put on weight is because we eat too much (apart from inherited tendencies). Thus the assumption for a long time was that people are too fat because they eat too much and do not have enough exercise. We have found this to be wrong.

In this chapter you will learn why this hypothesis is false. Above all you will understand that overweight can be traced back to an abnormal storage of energy, encouraged by metabolic processes, which, in turn, are triggered by an incorrect choice of food.

Furthermore, the explanation for weight gain lies in the height of the blood-sugar level and the formation of fat reserves that result from this. People, therefore, do not necessarily gain weight because they eat too much, but because they are eating the wrong way.

These somewhat theoretical explanations are necessary, however, so that we can know the real causes of weight gain. Only when we are really aware of these – in other words, when the scales fall from our eyes – can we be sure that we won't revert to the old pattern of behaviour and our old eating habits.

The hyperinsulinism trail

Since 1979 nutritionists have unambiguously highlighted the metabolic process in weight gain. They are agreed that in all cases of obesity, hyperinsulinism also occurs, regardless of the type or the mechanism. All the studies show that this hyperinsulinism is proportional to the excess weight.

This means that an obese person suffers much more severely from hyperinsulinism than a person who is only five or ten kilograms overweight. The conclusion to be drawn from this is that the main difference between overweight and slim people is that hyperinsulinism occurs in those who are overweight and not in those who are slim.

Let us imagine that two people live together and every day they eat exactly the same food containing an identical amount of energy. When, after several years, one of them is overweight and the other one is not, there can only be one reason: the overweight person suffers from hyperinsulinism and the slim one does not. In order to understand exactly what hyperinsulinism is, we must first know what insulin is.

In the previous chapter you learned that glycaemia means the glucose content (sugar content) in the blood. As we have already said, the normal glucose level with an empty stomach is around 1g per litre of blood.

As was explained earlier, glucose is the body's fuel. The blood acts as a permanent reservoir of glucose, from which the organs (brain, heart, kidneys, muscles) can meet their glucose requirements

The body has two possible ways of obtaining the necessary glucose and, at the same time, of maintaining the concentration at 1g per litre of blood.

The first way is to manufacture glucose. The body is able at all times to produce glucose from the fat reserves that are stored in the fatty tissues. When the need is very great, it is even possible for the body to produce glucose from the muscle mass, that is, from the proteins contained in the muscles.

The second way to obtain glucose is by the consumption of foods containing carbohydrates, i.e. all kinds of sugar, fruit and other starch products.

We know that carbohydrates are converted into glucose during digestion, with the exception of fructose. But before this can be stored in the body in the form of glycogen, glucose is transported through the blood. This means that after the consumption of carbohydrates, the resulting glucose causes a sudden rise in the blood-sugar level.

After the consumption of fruit, sweets or starch products, the concentration of blood sugar (which is normally 1g per litre of blood) increases suddenly. After fruit is eaten, for example, it is 1.20g, and 1.70g after potatoes are eaten. This sudden rise in the blood-sugar level after the absorption of carbohydrates is described as hyperglycaemia.

As soon as the threshold of 1g glucose per one litre of blood is greatly exceeded, we are in the realms of 'hyperglycaemia', i.e. the blood-sugar level is simply too high. If, on the other hand, the blood-sugar concentration drops too much (down to 0.50g/l), we speak of 'hypoglycaemia', in other words, the blood-sugar level is too low.

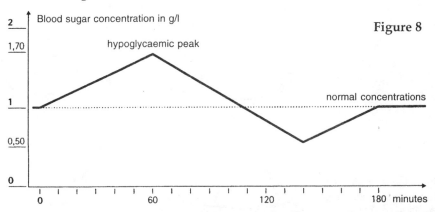

Figure 8

Hyperglycaemia depends on the glycaemic index of the carbohydrates consumed. Consequently, only slight hyperglycaemia occurs after fruit is eaten, which has a low glycaemic index (30). However, when sweets (with a glycaemic index of 75), or fried potatoes (with a glycaemic index of 95) are eaten, this leads to severe hyperglycaemia, which can, for example, reach 1.75g. In other words: if you eat too many sweets, you will make the blood-sugar level in your body rise.

Since the normal blood-sugar level is 1g/l, a mechanism to regulate it is triggered when the concentration is too high. Monitoring of this is carried out by an important organ, the pancreas, which releases the hormone insulin.

Insulin enables the release of glucose into the organs that need it, which brings about a decrease in the blood sugar level. Moreover – and this is really important – insulin encourages the formation of fat reserves.

As soon as the concentration of the blood-sugar level exceeds 1g/l, the pancreas releases insulin in order to restore normal conditions.

However, when the blood-sugar concentration falls below the normal measurement (hypoglycaemia), the body sees to it that the blood-sugar level rises again and once again restores the balance.

Normally the amount of insulin produced by the pancreas to lower the blood-sugar level has a direct ratio to the blood-sugar concentration.

For example, after the consumption of fruit, which triggers slight hyperglycaemia, the pancreas releases a small amount of insulin, since the blood-sugar level is only slightly raised.

65

FIRST EXPERIMENT:
100g white bread and
30g butter eaten

Figure 9

Representation of a blood
vessel
white bread ⇨ glucose
butter ⇨ fatty acids

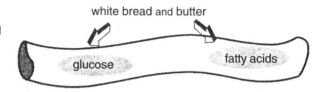

Figure 10

The glucose contained in
the blood triggers a high
secretion of insulin
(hyperinsulinism)

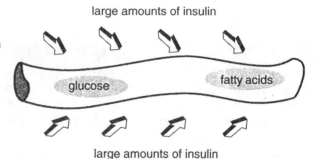

Figure 11

The insulin drives the
glucose out of the blood,
but as a large amount of
insulin remains, a large
amount of fatty acids is
excreted.

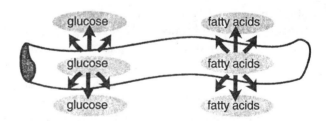

Figure 12

The glucose is stored as
glycogen.
The fatty acids are stored
in the fat reserves (weight
gain).

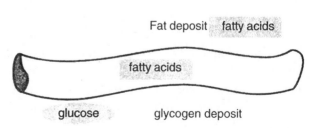

SECOND
EXPERIMENT
100g wholegrain bread
and 30g butter eaten

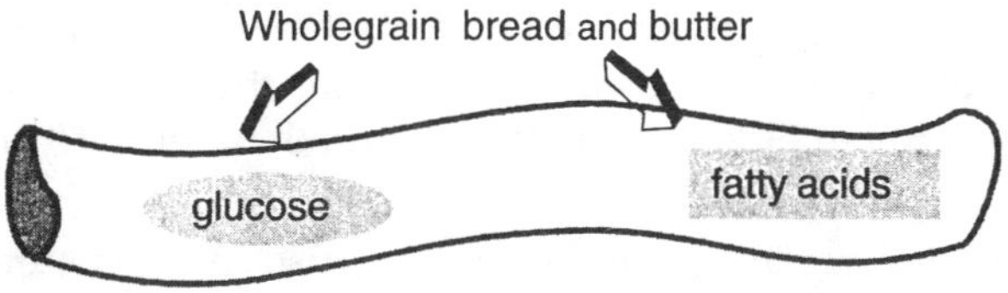

Wholegrain bread and butter

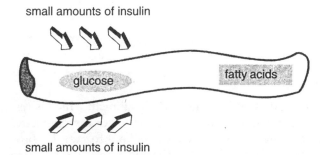

Figure 13

Depiction of a blood
vessel
wholegrain bread ⇨
glucose
butter ⇨fatty acids

small amounts of insulin

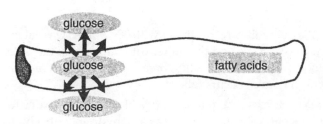

small amounts of insulin

Figure 14

The small quantity of
glucose triggers a very
low secretion of insulin.

Figure 15

The low insulin
secretion ensures
glucose is transported
from the blood, but is
not sufficient to excrete
fatty acids at the same
time.

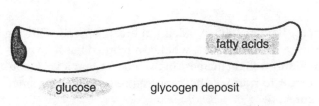

Figure 16

The glucose is stored
as glycogen.
The fatty acids are not
stored in the fat
reserves (no weight
gain).

glucose   glycogen deposit

However, after sweets have been eaten, which trigger severe hyperglycaemia, the pancreas secretes a large amount of insulin in order to bring the blood-sugar level back to normal.

In every case, the glucose that has been removed from the blood by insulin is either stored in the liver (as glycogen) or used by the organs that need it, for example the brain, kidneys or red blood corpuscles or stored under the form of fat as a reserve.

Our bodies are thus set up for a relative state of balance. Insulin contributes to this by compensating for an excess or a shortfall. Insulin is secreted by the pancreas. If the pancreas no longer functions properly, as a result of constant long-term stimulation, it releases a lot of insulin uncontrollably and this finally leads to the formation of fat reserves.

If you tend to be overweight, this can be put down to the fact that the function of the pancreas is disturbed. This means that if there is severe hyperglycaemia the pancreas will release an extremely large quantity of insulin. This is called 'hyperinsulinism'.

It has been proved scientifically that it is this hyperinsulinism which is responsible for the excessive formation of fat reserves. In order to understand this phenomenon better, two experiments were carried out to examine how the consumption of a slice of bread and butter affected a person tending to overweight.

First experiment

In the first experiment 100g of white bread, spread with 30g butter, was eaten. The bread is converted into glucose and the butter into fatty acids; they are transported via the blood (Figure 9). As white bread has a high glycaemic index (70), severe hyperglycaemia occurs (about 1.70g).

As a result, the pancreas releases a certain quantity of insulin, in order to lower the blood-sugar concentration again. Since a carbohydrate with a high glycaemic index is involved, an extremely high quantity of insulin is released (Figure 10). This hyperinsulinism leads to an excessive storage of part of the fatty acids from the butter (Figures 11 and 12).

Second experiment

In the second experiment, 100g of 100% wholegrain bread, spread with 30g of butter, was eaten (Figure 13). Since 100% wholegrain bread has a low glycaemic index (40), there is only a slight increase in the blood-sugar level (about 1.20g). In order to return it to normal, the pancreas releases a very small quantity of insulin (Figure 14).

Since no hyperinsulinism is caused when there is a low concentration of blood sugar, the pancreas only secretes the quantity of insulin needed to bring the slightly raised blood-sugar level back to normal (Figure 15).

The fatty acids in butter are not stored in excessive quantities, since the amount of insulin released is small (Figure 16).

These 'bread and butter experiments' show, although in a rather diagrammatic way, the mechanism of the formation of fat reserves, and thus weight gain, very clearly.

In both cases our 'guinea-pigs' ate the same: 100g bread and 30g butter. Why is there weight gain in the first case and not in the second? It is, of course, because of the composition of the bread! The combination of its nutrients is the only explanation.

White bread is a refined food. It not only lacks fibre but most proteins, vitamins, mineral salts and trace elements as well. For this reason it has a high glycaemic index. Hundred percent wholegrain bread, however, is a raw product which still contains all the nutrients and, especially, the fibre and proteins. It therefore has a low glycaemic index.

White bread triggers a sharp rise in the blood-sugar level and thus causes a weight increase through hyperinsulinism (storage of the fatty acids from butter). 100 % wholegrain bread causes a slight effect on the increase in blood sugar and only triggers a small release of insulin, so that no fatty acids from butter are stored.

This showed that it is not the energy (which is practically the same in both kinds of bread) contained in food that leads to weight gain. It is the composition of the food that has been eaten, that is, its nutrient content, which causes additional weight or not.

In the second experiment, there was, therefore, no weight gain, because the glycaemic index of the bread was low enough not to trigger hyperinsulinism, which is indirectly responsible for the production of extra pounds. It must be emphasised that there was no damage to pancreas function present in this case.

What differentiates a thin person from a fat one? If one of them (the fat one) puts on more weight than the other, although he eats the same (carbohydrates with a high glycaemic index), he will suffer from hyperinsulinism. In his case, the amount of insulin released is not in the right ratio to the amount of carbohydrate eaten. The thin person has no problem with this yet, perhaps, but it won't take long, if he goes on eating too many 'bad' carbohydrates.

Obesity is, therefore, only the indirect result of an excessive consumption of carbohydrates with a high glycaemic index (too much white sugar, white flour, potatoes) combined with an intake of fat.

Excessive consumption of 'bad' carbohydrates manifests itself in a permanently raised blood-sugar level, which causes extreme stimulation of the pancreas. Initially, the pancreas is able to withstand this stimulation, but after a few years it will show the first symptoms of weakness, as it is not designed for such an extreme situation. For this reason people will put on weight as they get older, because obesity always relates to the development of hyperinsulinism.

Because it is so essential. . .

Let us repeat this using other words, because it is so essential and important, in order to understand what is actually new about the Montignac Method:

- In hypoglycaemia, the hormone glucagon is released in the pancreas, which has the effect of resupplying the blood with glucose. Glucagon thus raises glycaemia. If glycaemia increases, as is the case after eating, and especially when this includes carbohydrates, the pancreas secretes the hormone insulin, which has the task of reducing glycaemia.

- Normally the amount of insulin necessary to lower the glycaemia to its normal level is proportional to the level of the glycaemia. In other words, if the glycaemia is slight, there will be a small insulin secretion; if the glycaemia is very high, the insulin secretion will be large.

This is exactly what happens with a slim person. The quantity of insulin secreted from the pancreas is always exactly proportional to the level of the glycaemia.

For those who are overweight, and obese people especially, things are different. As soon as the glycaemic peak is reached, the pancreas releases the insulin secretion. But now, instead of releasing the exact quantity into the blood that is needed to lower the glycaemia to its normal level, the pancreas releases a little too much, or much too much insulin.

When hyperinsulinism occurs, therefore, the pancreas releases a disproportionate amount of insulin in relation to the glycaemia.

It has been shown that hyperinsulinism is responsible for weight gain, as it triggers metabolic processes (lipogenesis), which means that the body stores part of the fats consumed at the last meal abnormally as fat reserves.

Without hyperinsulinism, fats stored in this way would have been converted differently in the metabolism. They would have been oxidised and the body would therefore have been able to make better use of them. This is why slim people are said to 'burn up' all the energy they consume, especially the fats.

Obese people, in contrast, tend rather to store up fats because of their hyper-insulinism and a possible insulin resistance. Hyperinsulinism is increased in obese people by a resistance to insulin. In reaction to hyperglycaemia, the pancreas secretes too much insulin. Although the quantity is too great, this is poorly recognised by the body, probably because the sensitivity of the receptors is defective.

Since the hyperglycaemia continues to be abnormal, the pancreas plays up and releases insulin again, which makes the hyperinsulinism even worse. A real vicious circle develops in which the hyperinsulinism intensifies the in-sulin resistance. As well as the formation of fat reserves, already familiar to us, there is an additional risk of reactive hyperglycaemia because of this in-sulin resistance.

Hyperinsulinism is, therefore, a disorder or disease of the metabolism. Fat and obese people have a more or less serious disorder of the pancreas.

When this was discovered at the beginning of the 1980s, scientists suspected (as most of them still do today) that hyperinsulinism was inherited; people had simply 'been unlucky'. For this reason, the only advice ever given to the obese was to lose weight. Scientists had discovered, you see, that hyperinsu-linism disappears with the pounds. Some of them concluded from this that hyperinsulinism is merely the result of overweight and obesity, which can be attributed to an excessive energy intake and to too little exercise.

All these 'experts' therefore came to the following simple conclusion: hyper-insulinism can only be controlled through weight loss, which can only hap-pen if the total calorie intake is reduced and physical activity is increased. A theory of hyperinsulinism, portrayed in such black and white terms, was not going to advance the cause of science very much.

The other hypothesis

On the basis of what I had discovered in diabetes research about the new division of carbohydrates according to their glycaemic index, I approached the problem from a different direction. Unlike those who thought that hy-perinsulinism was only a consequence of obesity, I put forward the hypothe-sis that it is obesity that is the consequence of hyperinsulinism.

From my own experience, too, I was able to draw the following conclusions:

- The consumption of carbohydrates with a **low glycaemic index stops weight gain** (and even leads to weight loss), because the cause of weight gain, hyperinsulinism, is reduced or eliminated

71

- **Obesity can only result from hyperinsulinism.**
- **Hyperinsulinism is the result of high levels of hyperglycaemia.** Hyperglycaemia is a result of an excessive consumption of carbohydrates with a high glycaemic index. This therefore means that the consumption of carbohydrates with a high glycaemic index indirectly (via hyperglycaemia and hyperinsulinism) leads to weight gain, because it encourages the storing of lipids. To a certain extent hyperinsulinism is the Trojan horse of lipids (fats) and the catalyst for obesity.
- In order to prevent overweight (or, rather, avoid it) it is sufficient to **change your eating habits** by eating the foods that have an exclusively low glycaemic index.

The glycaemic consequences of meals

Since the 1980s numerous studies on the glycaemic index have been carried out in the area of diabetes research. Thanks to this work we understand nowadays the various metabolic processes that result from our choice of carbohydrates. We know, therefore, that the glycaemic index of a carbohydrate can vary according to several parameters:

- **different types**: some types of rice (e.g. basmati rice) have a low index (50), whereas others (sticky rice) have a high index (70)
- **methods of preparation**: raw carrots have a low index (35), whereas the index of cooked carrots is high (85). The index of potatoes increases according to the method of preparation; 65, when they are boiled in their skins; 70, when they are peeled before boiling; 90 when they are pureed and 95 when they are roasted or deep-fat fried
- **industrial processing**: corn in its natural state has an index of 70, which rises to 85 after it has been processed to make cornflakes or popcorn. White pasta which is manufactured using high pressure like spaghetti has a low glycaemic index (40 to 45), whereas ravioli or macaroni, where high pressure is not used in production, have a high index
- **fibre and protein content**: lentils, which contain fibre (particularly of the soluble sort) and proteins have a very low glycaemic index (22 to 33) compared to other starchy foods like potatoes. Soya beans, which are high in protein, also have a very low glycaemic index.

A meal is complex in as far as it consists of different foods. Some foods can increase glycaemia; on the other hand, others contribute to its reduction.

What is important is the glycaemic total of the meal, for that will have a determining influence on hyperglycaemia after eating and thus, indirectly (if the hyperglycaemia level is high) on the hyperinsulinism responsible for abnormal formation of fat reserves as well.

Stay slim all our lives?
The deterioration in our eating habits

We have seen in the preceding chapters that gaining weight can be attributed to the consumption of carbohydrates with a high glycaemic index, which can lead to an abnormal storage of the ingested fats. We can now ask, with some justification, how it is that some people are able to eat carbohydrates with a high glycaemic index every day and still stay as thin as a rake. The answer is simple: their pancreas is (still) in a good condition and does not suffer from hyperinsulinism (yet).

So is it possible to stay slim all our lives, although we eat hyperglycaemially? It is actually possible but, as we shall see, more and more unlikely.

Some people can stay slim all their lives in spite of bad eating habits. This means that they have had a pancreas that has functioned very well since the day they were born and which can defend itself against the 'bad' carbohydrates all through their life, so that hyperinsulinism does not occur.

Other people (the majority) have a pancreas which functions well initially; thanks to this they stay slim for a long time in spite of bad eating habits. And then, at 30, 35 or – especially – after 40, they put on weight. Some will become obese in their old age and develop diabetes.

This means that their pancreas has put up a good fight over several decades but has finally 'given up the ghost', because it has been overloaded day after day, year after year, in its struggle against hyperglycaemic attacks. Rather like an engine, constantly mistreated, which gradually functions less and less efficiently.

And then there are those (Michel Montignac is one of them) who came into the world with a pancreas that was already malfunctioning. This is why heredity is always automatically blamed for a weakness like this.

It is a fact that children with obese parents (who therefore suffer from hyperinsulinism) are much more likely to have a weak pancreas. This is almost always the case when they have been fed in a hyperglycaemic way from early childhood.

In 1997 the World Health Organisation warned against a worldwide epidemic of obesity. In the same year an extensive study in the United States showed that the number of obese people had paradoxically risen by 33% in the previous ten years, although during the same period the average energy intake was reduced, fat consumption dropped by 11% and the number of consumers of reduced calorie products rose from 19% to 76%.

This survey shows clearly that weight gain does not depend on calorie intake, since this has dropped considerably. Increasing obesity is more attributable to the declining nutritional value of modern food.

If you study the glycaemic index table (Table 2) closely you will find that all the foods in the left-hand column have a high glycaemic index and that they are all foods which have been refined (sugar, flour, white rice), processed industrially (cornflakes, puffed rice, modified starch, chocolate bars) or that they are 'new' foods, potatoes, for example, or white flour or sugar which have been used for less than two hundred years.

It is exactly these foods that are preferred nowadays in most Western industrialised countries and which, in the course of globalisation, are increasingly being eaten in other countries.

If, on the other hand, you look at the right-hand column of the table, with the low glycaemic indices, you will find that most of the foods listed there are scarcely eaten any more today or are eaten increasingly rarely (wholegrain bread, wholegrain cereal, high-fibre flour, wholegrain rice, lentils, dried beans, dried peas, chick peas…) or are not eaten in sufficient quantities (fruit, green vegetables).

All these foods were regularly on the menu fifty years ago.

We have to realise, therefore, that the food people ate in the past (up to a few decades ago) mostly consisted of foods with a low glycaemic index, which therefore had a low glycaemic effect. The glycaemic consequences of meals were insignificant; our forefathers had a pancreas that had fewer demands on it, so the risk of hyperinsulinism was small.

For thousands of years, our way of eating has stayed relatively the same. It was only at the beginning of the twentieth century that eating habits in the industrialised countries in the West deteriorated drastically. Little by little we have gone from a low-glycaemic diet to a high one.

Under the influence of an increasingly hyperglycaemic way of eating, our contemporaries' pancreas has come under more and more stress and has reacted by increasing hyperinsulinism; this has finally led to a situation where there are ever more fat and obese people.

Let us look at the main components, for example, of the American way of eating, which by now mostly consists of fast food. They are:

- **low-fibre white flour** (index 95), which is used for hamburgers, hot dogs sandwiches, biscuits, crackers etc.
- **sugar**, which occurs in industrial products (canned foods, mustard, ketchup, crackers, biscuits, ready-prepared meal. . .) and drinks (lemonades, fruit juices, iced tea, Coca Cola. . .)
- **corn** (index 70), which is eaten unprocessed or processed for use in cornflakes or popcorn (index 85)
- **white rice** (high-yield, index 70), or processed as puffed rice (index 85) or rice pudding (index 85)

Apart from these, Americans prefer beer (index 110) and ready-prepared meals containing glucose syrup (index 100), maltodextrin (100) and modified starch (95). You can draw the conclusion from this that there is a close relationship between the American diet and the metabolic illnesses that indirectly result from it: obesity and diabetes.

The problem of obesity, recognised nowadays in the Western world, must be taken seriously. It has arisen because, for roughly fifty years, our food has contained too many 'bad' carbohydrates. This change in our eating habits began almost one hundred and fifty years ago when new foods with a hyperglycaemic effect spread throughout the Western world in the first half of the nineteenth century. These foods were sugar, potatoes and white flour.

Sugar

Until the sixteenth century sugar was virtually unknown in the Western world. It was occasionally used as a flavouring, but since its scarcity made it very expensive, it was only available to the extremely wealthy.

The discovery of the New World made a partial spread of sugar cane possible, but because of the transport and refining costs sugar still remained a luxury article for the rich.

In 1780 sugar consumption was less than one kilo per year per person. Not until the discovery of sugar extraction from beet in 1812 did the prime costs decrease permanently and because of this sugar gradually became a popular consumer product. Statistics concerning sugar consumption in France show the following figures in kilos per year per person:

- 1800: 0.6
- 1965: 40
- 1880: 8
- 1990: 35
- 1900: 17
- 1930: 30

Sugar is known to be a carbohydrate with a high glycaemic index (75). As a result, its consumption triggers a hyperglycaemic attack, which results in an excessive stimulation of the pancreas.

Happily, sugar consumption by the French is (still) the lowest in the Western world. The English consume 49 kilos, the Germans 52 kilos and the world record is held by the Americans with 63 kilos per year per person!

Potatoes

Quite a few people believe that the potato is part of the legacy of old Europe. That is not so, for it only spread gradually in the eighteenth century. Since its discovery in Peru in the middle of the sixteenth century it was simply used as pig food. Moreover, that's what it was called, and people were very suspicious of it as it was part of the solanum family, which were mostly poisonous.

It must be emphasised that the potato has the highest glycaemic index; fried potatoes, for example, have a higher glycaemic index than sugar.

The way potatoes are prepared also plays an extremely important role, since starches, which vary in their resistance to digestion, are formed in the process. The resulting amount of digestion-resistant starch is so small in fried or mashed potatoes that most of them are digested.

Moreover, potatoes are of little use as far as nutrition is concerned, since, alongside the powerful effect they have in increasing blood sugar when cooked, they only have a very low nutritional value (8mg/100 vitamin C and a small amount of fibre). Their vitamin, mineral and trace element content is all the more valueless as these nutrients are in the skin and so are automatically removed when the potatoes are peeled.

Lengthy storage of potatoes also reduces their vitamin content.

Flour

Flour has always been sieved or sifted. In the past it was sifted coarsely by hand and, because of the high price of prime costs (30% matter removed), fine flour was only accessible to a few rich people. Since ordinary people had to make do with black bread, white bread became one of the symbolic principal demands of the French Revolution.

Only with the discovery of the cylinder mill in 1870 did it become possible to reduce the prime costs for grinding flour substantially and to offer white bread for sale daily in considerably larger quantities. As we know, however, nutrients (i.e. proteins), essential fatty acids, vitamins, mineral salts, trace elements and fibre, were removed from the flour when it was ground. As we also know, grinding wheat flour causes the glycaemic index to increase from 40 to 70, and as a result it becomes a food that has a hyperglycaemic effect.

Nowadays we eat less bread than a hundred years ago perhaps, but in exchange we take in more white flour through the consumption of pasta, rolls, pizza, biscuits, various cakes. . .

As everyone knows, rice comes from Asia, where the locals usually eat it together with vegetables that are rich in fibre, vitamins, mineral salts and trace elements, which weaken the glycaemic effect. In the West, where rice is processed, we prefer to eat it with meat that does not contain fibre but saturated fatty acids instead.

Moreover, it should be emphasised that genuine Asiatic rice such as basmati (even when it is white) has a much lower glycaemic index than Western rice, which comes from high-yield types. At all events, rice is the fourth carbohydrate with a high glycaemic index to have become an integral part of our modern food intake recently.

Corn

The same is true of corn, which is found in the West in the form of hybrid plants that have been developed in the laboratory to increase yield.

The original corn on which the Indians lived has a much lower glycaemic index (roughly 30). As has been shown, this is because of the larger amount of soluble fibre. This high soluble-fibre content not only creates a low blood-sugar level but also makes possible the storage of moisture.

Because of the soluble fibre that is lacking, it is necessary nowadays to irrigate modern corn, which leads to a fall in ground water.

Carrots

Starch in carrots, like that in potatoes, is particularly sensitive to heat. That is why cooked carrots are 'bad' carbohydrates and raw carrots are 'good' carbohydrates. Raw carrots have a very low glycaemic index of 35 and are only to be recommended in this form. Starch is destroyed by cooking, leading to a sharp rise in the potential for hyperglycaemia. The glycaemic index is 85. If you would like to lose weight, you should not eat cooked carrots.

Paradoxically, people lose weight when they eat raw carrots, especially if they are grated or in a salad. In contrast to potatoes, raw carrots are easy to digest.

Pasta

Pasta is made from white flour, as you know. For this reason, you will probably expect us to advise you against it. You will, I'm sure, be surprised to learn that this is not so. Over the years it has been established that there are at least some sorts that not only do not make you fat, they even help you to lose weight. This needs to be explained in more detail.

The first thing you need to know is that genuine pasta must consist of hard wheat, whereas bread is made from soft wheat. The difference is that hard wheat contains more protein and fibre (even low-fibre flour) and this contributes to the lowering of the glycaemic index.

You also need to know that some types of pasta (especially spaghetti) is 'pastificised'. Pastification involves a mechanical process in which the pasta is 'extruded' under high pressure. A protective layer around the pasta is formed in this process that reduces the gelling of the starch during cooking, provided that the cooking time is as short as possible (*al dente* as the Italians say), in other words, four to six minutes at most.

White pastificised pasta (spaghetti) with an average cooking time (eight to twelve minutes) has a low glycaemic index (50) because of the properties of hard wheat and the pastification process. If the cooking time is longer (twelve to sixteen minutes), the glycaemic index will rise to 55. If the cooking time is shorter (five to six minutes), the glycaemic index is much lower (45). Cooling pasta reduces the glycaemic index again (degeneration of starch). Thus, pastificised hard wheat spaghetti, cooked *al dente*, has a glycaemic index of 40 when it is eaten cold (e.g. as a salad).

With wholewheat pasta, under the conditions mentioned above, the glycaemic index is about another five points lower.

What we have said above, however, does not apply to pasta made from soft wheat and applies even less to pasta that has not been pastificised, for example ribbon noodles, macaroni, lasagne and ravioli.

You therefore need to be particularly careful in your choice of pasta. In some countries like France, the pasta manufacturers have to use hard wheat. That is not the case in the countries of northern Europe. There, pasta made of soft wheat is often on sale. Moreover, it is not easy to check if the pasta has been pastificised, since the manufacturer is not obliged to give this information on the packaging. Spaghetti is always pastificised.

Tagliatelle, on the other hand, is not pastificised systematically. The thinner it is (if it has been industrially produced), the more likely it is to have been pastificised. Beware of fresh pasta, available in a good many restaurants, as it is not pastificised but produced using a small machine, which cuts out narrow strips from home-made pasta dough (similar to pizza dough).

Fine Chinese noodles, on the other hand, which are made from soya flour (or mung beans) with a very low glycaemic index, can be recommended. Since they are also pastificised and only cooked for a very short time they are the ultimate among 'noodles' with a low glycaemic index.

So, become accustomed to eating spaghetti (as thin as possible) *al dente* with various sauces (tomato, mushroom, or curry sauce) or in a salad (as a starter).

Pulses

Some pulses can contribute to weight loss. These include dried beans, chick-peas and, especially, lentils. Green lentils and dried peas have an even lower index, 22, than green beans.

Fruit

Fruit is a sacred cow. If we dared to recommend crossing it off our eating plan, many of you would close the book at this point from sheer outrage. For fruit is a symbol in our culture. It stands for vitality, abundance and health. For your peace of mind we will not leave out fruit, as it is irreplaceable. We just need to eat it in a different way to make use of all its advantages and, at the same time avoid its disadvantages (flatulence).

Fruit contains carbohydrates (glucose, sucrose and, especially, fructose), and it also contains fibre, which lowers the glycaemic index and thus reduces the absorption of sugar. Apples and pears contain a particularly large amount of pectin (soluble fibre) with which the rise in glycaemia can be restricted. The energy from fruit can be simply used by the muscles and is therefore scarcely ever stored as fat reserves. (Fresh) fruit, however, should preferably be eaten on an empty stomach. This advice has more to do with digestion than with weight loss. You see, if you eat fruit at the end of the meal as usual, you may have problems with your digestion. Older people in particular are especially susceptible to this; children are a great deal less so. Where adults are concerned, everything depends on how susceptible you are individually. What is the reason for this?

Digestion begins with chewing in the mouth and ends in the small intestine. Fruit, therefore, should pass through the stomach quickly.

If fruit is eaten after foods like meat or cheese, which contain lipids and proteins, its passage through the stomach will be blocked until the lipids and proteins have been digested, although it ought actually to move quickly into the intestine. The fruit will, in consequence, be trapped in the stomach and will begin to ferment in this warm, damp environment; there may even be a slight formation of alcohol. The whole process of digestion can suffer as a result (flatulence).

Fruit must therefore be eaten neat! This rule should perhaps be learnt in school, although children's bodies are able to react better. Adults, especially the elderly, should eat no fruit at the end of a meal.

So, when should it be eaten?

Whenever you have not eaten: in the mornings, for example, before breakfast. You should wait fifteen minutes before eating anything else, so that the fruit can pass through the stomach undisturbed. You can also eat some fruit late in the evening before going to bed, at least three hours after finishing supper. You can eat a piece of fruit in the afternoon too, provided you have a long enough time gap after lunch or before supper.

However, since every rule has its exception, there are also exceptions for different sorts of fruits, where there is almost no likelihood of fermentation because of their low sugar concentration. This is the case with strawberries, raspberries, blackberries, redcurrants and blueberries, which you can eat at the end of a meal without any problems.

You can also eat fruit when it has been cooked at the end of a meal, as it no longer ferments in the stomach. Do not forget, however, that most of the vitamin C is lost in cooking. Lemons do not ferment either; you can drink lemon juice (unsweetened) at any time or use it for seasoning (on fish or in salad dressings).

Whenever possible you should eat fruit unpeeled, after you have washed it thoroughly. The peel contains a lot of fibre and, often, the highest concentration of vitamins. The added advantage of eating the peel with the fruit is that the fruit's glycaemic index is further reduced. You will improve your weight loss if you follow this rule.

Drinks, especially alcoholic ones, also come under the heading of important foods.

Alcoholic drinks

Alcohol makes you fat! You believe this because it's what you've been told. You have perhaps even been talked into having a guilty conscience because the alcohol you drink regularly has been blamed for all those extra pounds. We would like to try to settle this question objectively.

It is true that alcohol can contribute to weight gain if it is drunk in excessive amounts. But if you practise moderation, it can be neutral. In your weight-loss phase, you should restrict your alcohol consumption to a small glass (10cl), to be drunk at the end of the meal. If you want to play safe, you should go without this small symbolic amount as well, so as not to be tempted to drink more. We will see that it will be possible to drink two or three glasses of wine a day without a second thought after you have lost weight, without putting weight on again.

Alcohol provides energy that is used by the body as a matter of priority. During this time the body will therefore tend not to make use of its fat reserves as fuel. Weight loss will be halted. This is particularly so when you have not eaten.

If the stomach is already full, especially with fat and proteins (meat, fish, cheese), alcohol will take a lot longer to pass through the body and will contribute less to the formation of fat reserves as it does so. On the other hand, you will have to give up your aperitif. If you absolutely have to drink with your guests, choose a non-alcoholic drink like tomato juice or mineral water.

If it is not possible to do anything else, then accept a glass of champagne as an aperitif, but whatever you do, do not drink it on an empty stomach. Have a few nibbles to start with. You will soon learn to recognise the right ones. On the forbidden list are crisps, savoury biscuits, and canapés on toast. Allowed are olives, cheese, certain types of sausage (for example, dried salami) or fish (e.g. smoked). Two or three cubes of cheese or one slice of sausage will be enough to close the pylorus (the sphincter muscle between the stomach and the small intestine) and so delay the passage of alcohol into the bloodstream.

In the first phase of weight loss you should, however, try to do without your aperitif completely, since in this phase the basic rules of the Method should be applied consistently in order to guarantee an effective weight loss.

Digestifs

Say goodbye to all spirits. Brandies and many types of after-dinner liqueurs are delicious (if they agree with you) but in every respect they are bad for your figure. Perhaps you value digestifs highly, but only because of the helpful effect they are supposed to have on your digestion. Bear in mind that, even after a sumptuous repast, you will no longer have any digestive problems when you follow the nutritional principles described in this book.

Beer

Beer is another drink that should only be enjoyed in small amounts. Its side-effects are all too well-known; bloating, weight gain (especially when it is drunk outside mealtimes), bad breath, digestive disorders in spite of the work of diastase (an important enzyme, whose function is to activate the digestion). You need to be careful with beer, since it contains alcohol and, especially, a carbohydrate (maltose) that has a very high glycaemic index (110).

In addition, the combination of alcohol and sugar encourages the occurrence of hypoglycaemia, a cause of fatigue and, therefore, reduced energy. If, up to now, you have drunk a lot of beer, you should severely restrict your consumption, especially outside mealtimes. During meals you can perhaps drink 20cl maximum but you need to know that you would lose weight more efficiently if you were prepared to give it up.

Wine

We have already talked about wine, but there are still a lot of interesting things to say about it, which we will do in a later chapter. Since the beginning of the 1980s many scientific studies have shown that wine (especially red wine) has indisputable qualities that promote and protect health. A moderate but regular consumption of wine can lower the risk of cardiovascular diseases. Moreover, the risk of heart attacks is reduced among wine drinkers.

In 1995 there was verification that the beneficial effect of wine can be attributed particularly to the antioxidants it contains: the highly effective polyphenols. It was even proved that, with a moderate wine consumption, some of these polyphenols could act as a preventive against certain types of cancers and even Alzheimer's disease. What interests us particularly here, however, is whether consumption of wine leads to weight gain.

We have already said that excessive wine or alcohol consumption can make you fat. Two or three glasses, on the other hand, have a more or less neutral effect. A small glass of wine (10cl) at the end of the meal might even have positive effects on insulin secretion, in the opinion of some experts.

If you have sufficient willpower to stick to these small amounts, the effectiveness of your weight loss will be increased. If that is not the case, you would be better to give up wine for the whole of the weight-loss period.

We will also see that later on, when you are in the process of stabilising your weight, you will be able to drink wine without it affecting your weight adversely. Wine consumption, however, must be skilfully co-ordinated with the carbohydrates you eat. If you are still in the process of losing weight, you should stick to the advice that has been given, even if you find it difficult to join in a family party or a meeting with friends without having a drop of wine to drink. If you actually announce that you are not drinking, it can be awkward for the others. For that reason, do as follows: let your glass be filled and reach for it as if you were going to drink normally. Moisten your lips instead of drinking. In short, pretend, which is not easy. But if you do it skilfully, nobody will notice that you haven't 'joined in'. You can deal with the bread in the same way. To do so, take a piece of bread but leave it crumbled on the table. You can ignore the amount of alcohol contained in wine vinegar. You can, therefore, use it to season raw food and salads, unless you prefer to use a lemon.

Coffee

Many people think that aromatic Italian espresso does the most harm. They are wrong, as the caffeine content is not necessarily higher but the taste is more intense, because of the pressure used in its preparation. Filter coffee is much more dubious. Even when it is supposedly weak, it contains a lot of caffeine.

For your weight-loss programme to succeed, you must create the optimal conditions. In this context you need to know that although coffee contains no 'bad' carbohydrates, it can lead to a slight increase in insulin secretion, especially in people who suffer from severe hyperinsulinism. Therefore the recommendation is to restrict coffee consumption and give it up completely at the beginning.

If you drink a lot of strong coffee, it is almost certainly because you would like its stimulating effect to make you feel more wide-awake. If you regularly experience an energy low around eleven in the morning or when you are digesting in the afternoon it is because you are reacting hypoglycaemically. In that case, drink decaffeinated coffee or pure Arabica coffee, which contains much less caffeine.

Like smoking and drinking, strong coffee consumption is a form of addiction that has developed over the course of the years. If it agrees with you, why not? If it doesn't you should give it up. To lose weight properly you should use your willpower for all your other goals.

Once you have reached your goal and your pancreas is functioning properly again, you can round off your meal occasionally with a good espresso.

Lemonade and soft drinks

These drinks are almost always manufactured from synthetic fruit or plant extracts and all have the same big disadvantage; they contain a lot of sugar (GI=70). They should, therefore, be avoided because of their high sugar content, especially as the artificial carbonic acid they contain can lead to aerophagia (chronic gulping of air) in susceptible people.

Worst of all are cola drinks, which need to be banned or specially labelled like cigarette packets: 'This product will endanger your health.' It is very regrettable, at any rate, that the consumption of cola drinks has risen so sharply worldwide.

Here we will quote Doctor Emile-Gaston Peeters, who had the following to say on the subject:

'At the present time the so-called cola drinks on the European market contain per 19cl (content of a small bottle) roughly 21mg of caffeine and 102mg of phosphoric acid. Caffeine acts as very strong stimulant. Phosphoric acid is extremely acidic and there is a risk that the balance of calcium and phosphorus in the bloodstream will be disturbed because of the high concentration of phosphorus and this can lead to a serious lack of calcium in the bones. Finally, we would have to be sure that the phosphoric acid used did not contain any excessive traces of toxic heavy metals. The conclusion is simple: children and young people must be expressly warned against drinking so-called cola drinks in their present form. They are not good for anyone.'

It may be hard, but it applies equally to children and adults: no lemonade, no soft drinks and, above all, no cola drinks.

Milk

Whole milk is a complex drink, as it contains protein, carbohydrates (lactose) and fats. We will also see later that milk fats (saturated) are bad. For this reason you should preferably use skimmed milk. You can also use powdered milk in a higher measure than the one given so that you get a cream-like high-protein liquid that will assist the weight-loss process.

Low-fat quark, which is very healthy because of its high protein and low carbohydrate content (5g per 100g), is also to be recommended. You should always use quark that has been drained so that you ingest as little lactose (whey) as possible. You should also avoid cream-like, stirred quark preparations that have been industrially homogenised. The best milk product is yoghurt (non-fat or low-fat), which is very healthy, on account of its milk enzymes.

Fruit juices

What we said above about fruit also applies to fresh fruit juices; that means juices that have been squeezed immediately before use.

However, fruit juices have a higher glycaemic index than the fruits from which they are made, for the simple reason that they contain no pulp, that is, fibre. For this reason, fruit juice (apart from lemon juice) can increase glycaemia. In your weight-loss phase, you should therefore preferably eat fruit.

Normal commercial fruit juices, even those with 100% fruit content and no sugar, have far fewer vitamins and fibre than freshly squeezed fruit juice. They also contain too much acid. They should therefore only be drunk occasionally.

How fat are you?
How to calculate your ideal weight

At the moment there are two methods given in most textbooks for calculating your ideal weight.

1. The Lorentz Formula

For women: weight = ((height-1) – ((height-1.4)/2))*100

For men: weight = ((height-1) – ((height-1.5)/4))*100

This kind of calculation, however, has the disadvantage that it does not take age or bone weight into account. It is therefore unsuitable for small women (1.50m). You should therefore take into account the weight you feel happiest with.

The second method is the so-called BMI.

2. BMI (Body Mass Index)

This is an internationally recognised formula that makes an extremely exact definition of body weight possible. This formula gives the ratio between the weight (in kilos) and the height (in metres squared):

$$BMI = \frac{weight\ (kg)}{(height \times height)\ (m)}$$

You can determine your own BMI with the aid of the following information:

- BMI between 20 and 23: normal body weight
- BMI between 24 and 29: overweight
- BMI over 30: obesity

In contrast to the Lorentz formula the normal body weight can fluctuate within a specific range according to the Body Mass Index and is not fixed to an exact measurement.

Distribution of fats

Paradoxically, the scales are not always the best means of ascertaining if you are overweight, as the body weight usually consists of bones, muscles, innards, water and fat.

Adiposity, or obesity, is merely defined as an excess of fat. In women the fat mass forms roughly 25% of the body weight. If sportsmen or sportswomen weigh rather more on the scales they are not necessarily to be described as fat, since this extra body weight can be mainly attributed to a greater muscle mass.

Water, which makes up two thirds of body weight alone, can easily cause weight fluctuations (one or two kilos).

'Slimming' and 'losing weight' are therefore two quite different things: slimming means losing excessive fat, whereas you may lose weight when there is merely a water loss. For this reason it is absolutely pointless to take diuretics when you want to slim, quite apart from their hidden risks.

Definition of the fat mass

Nowadays it is possible to define fat mass exactly: you are attached to a machine (as with an electrocardiogram) and water, muscle and fat mass will become visible on a monitor.

With this machine the fat mass can be measured exactly and its alteration during the slimming phase observed. Unfortunately, up to now, only very few nutritional specialists have such equipment at their disposal. Moreover, this machine only highlights the quantity of fat and gives no indication of the distribution of the fat mass in the body. This could be achieved with a scanner, for example, or by measuring the abdomen round the navel and then round the hips to find the ratio between them, which should be less than 0.85. A description of the different kinds of obesity follows.

Obesity in men

With male obesity, the fat deposits mostly in the upper half of the body (face, neck, chest, abdomen above the navel).

This excess weight often leads to certain metabolic disorders; diabetes, high blood pressure, hyperinsulinism, hypercholesterolaemia, hypertriglyceridaemia, cardiovascular diseases. . .

In this kind of obesity, the fat cells (adipose cells) are extremely enlarged because of an excess of fat, but the number of cells does not usually increase. In this case it is relatively easy to lose weight.

Obesity in women

When the fat mass is predominantly in the lower part of the body (abdomen, hips, upper thighs, bottom), we speak of 'female obesity'. In this form, the metabolic disorders mentioned above rarely occur. Vein weaknesses or arthritis of the knee or hips may often be observed, however. The damage is of two kinds, both physical and aesthetic; especially as for women in this category cellulite often occurs too.

Deep fat deposits

This third kind of obesity was only discovered recently. It is an excess of abdominal fats in the innards. This deep fat deposit, which can often not be seen from the outside (for this reason waist size looks quite normal), nevertheless presents a risk as it can encourage diabetes or cardiovascular diseases.

Smokers, male and female, are particularly prone to these deep fat deposits, which can accompany a normal bodyweight.

Setting realistic goals

Even if scales don't help you to find out exactly how overweight you are, they are still most frequently used to establish what weight loss you have already achieved.

But you must set yourself a realistic goal! A fifty-year-old man or woman cannot expect to reach the weight they were when they were twenty again, especially as weight loss is likelier to be successful if you set yourself a realistic target rather than a standard which is much too high.

But before you attempt to lose weight, you need to ask yourself why you actually want to slim. Afterwards will you accept the new way you look? Because sometimes, when people are suddenly concerned with their weight, there is another problem in the background, marital or family squabbles, for example.

In addition, a necessity to lose weight does not always exist. Many people, for example, suffer from psychological problems that find their expression in weight loss. For others, overweight provides a sort of protective wall that they erect against their fellow human beings. With women this is sometimes directed against men, because they are resisting being desired sexually. It is clear that a self-diagnosis becomes difficult in such a case. However, if you think long and hard about it, you might find the cause. Even if not everyone feels the need to slim, it is no bad thing to alter bad eating habits.

Especially important!

Also, if you feel unable to complete Phase I (which is aimed at a considerable weight loss), absolutely all that is needed is to apply the basic principles of the Method (Phase II). By doing so, there will not only be a physical alteration that will gradually become clearer and clearer, there will also be a conclusive change in the way that you eat, which will eventually benefit your health (both from a physical and an emotional point of view).

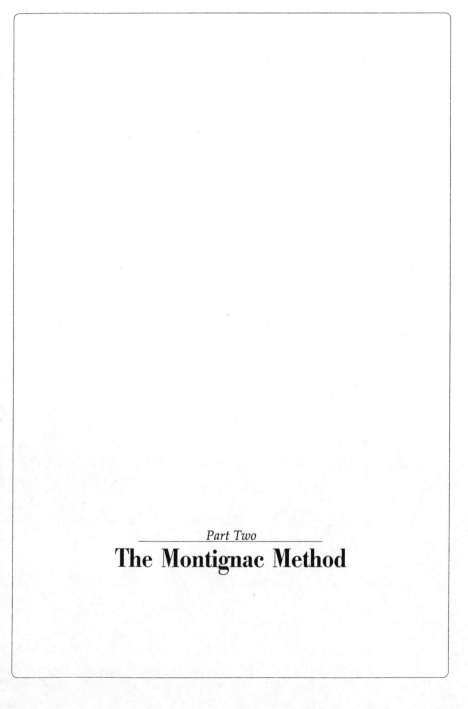

Part Two

The Montignac Method

Phase I: Losing weight with the Montignac Method

Basically it is easy to reduce your weight with the Montignac Method. You simply limit yourself to foods with a low glycaemic index.

But in order to recognise this simple thing we need to learn to free ourselves from the things we have mislearned, for often ideas that have been passed down to us are so firmly fixed in our subconscious that they are tantamount to cultural conditioning. The simple thoughts and the elementary scientific principles developed here have, unfortunately, only met with approval in very few doctors' surgeries. You must not rely, therefore, on those around you supporting you in your plan.

So now here we are in Phase I of the Montignac Method, and we want to reduce our weight. When we speak of Phase I, it presupposes that there is a Phase II.

Phase II is the phase following our successful weight loss and will help us to maintain our weight so that we do not fall into the so-called 'yo-yo' diet trap, i.e. putting on more weight after a phase of weight reduction than before. We must avoid that.

- Phase I is the weight loss phase
- Phase II is called the stabilisation phase

If you want to carry through a project as ambitious as reducing your own bodyweight, you need first of all to set yourself a target.

Using a really simple method, determine what BMI (Body Mass Index) you have and then establish how many surplus pounds you would like to lose. As you do so, take into account that every person is an individual and include also age, sex, and character, as well as your eating habits and diets in the past.

For these reasons it is difficult to say how much you will lose each week. For some one kilo is a lot, for others it will be more. Many slim down quickly at the beginning and then slow down. Don't be worried. Don't forget that everyone here must be looked at individually.

Tackle this in a positive but determined way. Don't think of the pounds but imagine your ideal weight. See your target and simply go for it, whoops, simply eat your way to it in accordance with the Montignac Method.

At the same time you need to pay attention to the fundamental metabolic processes that you learned about in the previous chapters. On the other hand, to be as effective as possible, you also need to apply a few rules that are a matter of sound common sense.

One of the rules says that you should not miss any meals (especially not lunch), because otherwise the body tends to form abnormal fat reserves at the following meal.

You should therefore allow for three meals a day and possibly a snack in the afternoon. You should have a substantial breakfast, a normal lunch and a light supper. The reason for this is that one and the same meal makes you fatter in the evening than in the morning, especially if it is fatty. Carrying through Phase I depends on one principle, which is the foundation of the Method, and on two rules:

⇨ **Fundamentalprinciple:** select your foods in such a way that the glycaemic total at the end of the meal is as low as possible and the insulin reaction is therefore kept to the minimum.

⇨ **Rules: two meal types are possible:**

- a fast and protein meal (lipoprotein) (e.g. meat or fish) with carbohydrates with a very low glycaemic index, such as green lentils, chick peas, green vegetables, equal to or below 35, or

- a carbohydrate-protein meal with no saturated fats and optionally with a small amount of monounsaturated or polyunsaturated fats. The glycaemic index of the carbohydrates must be below 50

So much for the broad picture at the beginning. Let us now deal with the method in Phase I.

The Montignac Method in Phase I

Looking at television advertisements for food, it is striking how differently they are done depending on whether they are about food for animals or humans.

In the case of animal food, the advertising message is presented in a fairly classical way. First of all, you see an animal breeder, as involving an expert always makes things more significant. Then a close-up follows of the animal, a dog perhaps, running around freely to emphasise how much energy it has. Next, our attention is drawn to its beautiful coat and the lively look in its eyes, which indicate its excellent state of health.

Finally, a vet comes into view and explains that this animal is in such a remarkable condition because his master feeds him on Product X; he vouches for its quality. There then follows a list of all the indispensable nutrients contained in the food, such as proteins, vitamins, mineral salts, trace elements and fibre.

A commercial extolling the advantages of food for human beings is made quite differently. The price, the packaging or its keeping qualities will nearly always be in the forefront.

A cyclist is late arriving, for example, and his fellow cyclists have finished off the soup in an obviously self-centred manner. They calm him down, for with an instant soup – and the brand is recommended afterwards – he can make himself soup 'just like it used to be' in a matter of seconds.

This is obviously a product substitute, where no one would dream of questioning its ingredients (sodium glutamate, sugar, modified starch, preservatives. . .), never mind show any interest in the absence of almost all nutrients.

When making commercials, the advertising man will always seize on sensitive topics and make use of symbols that influence the viewers' subconscious.

Why should anyone mention the nutrient content of a food in order to extol its advantages if noone is responsive to it, and on top of that, noone is interested?

For almost half a century the significance that food can have for health and the preservation of life has gradually been forgotten in our society. Since nutritional experts were obsessed with the energy aspects of foods, the food industry was able to concentrate completely on economic objectives; this has led to a massive technological development.

A change has taken place in the way we think; people's relationship to food has gradually altered as a result of urbanisation, the structure of society, working women and leisure time. We must beware of reducing eating to a gratification of a physiological need. People have to eat something of necessity in the same way they go to the lavatory. Under these circumstances, people naturally don't see why they should have to pay a lot of money for food. For this reason, the choice of food depends first and foremost on the price. Fast-food restaurants have reacted accordingly.

Most Romance countries like France, Italy or Spain have a different attitude to food. For them, food plays quite a different role. Eating is almost a ritual. Even though it helps to support life, food is a pleasure, since it is looked at from a hedonistic viewpoint.

The gourmet and cooking tradition in Mediterranean countries is not just a popular custom but also a fundamental element of their culture. With its differences, idiosyncrasies and geographical peculiarities, this tradition constitutes a real skill.

In consequence, lunchtime is sacred and is kept free. In the provinces offices, shops and local administration buildings are closed; most people go home and eat lunch with the family. Others meet in the cafeteria or the canteen. Lunch is one of life's important ceremonies and is organised according to definite rules.

Eating is a symbol of the best things in life. For this reason people take time with their food and spend money on it gladly.

The French paradox

We have already mentioned this paradox. But how can it help us in Phase I? Now, on 17 November 1991, the well-known American television programme 'Sixty Minutes' broadcast a twenty-minute piece with the title 'The French Paradox'. The report said that the French were in a significantly better state of health than the Americans, although they spent a lot of time on food, ate 30% more fat, did not exercise and drank ten times more wine.

The average weight of a Frenchman is the lowest in the whole of the Western world and the mortality rate from cardiovascular illnesses is the lowest after Japan. The CBS broadcast referred to findings that had been gathered by the World Health Organisation within the framework of an investigation (called 'Monica').

How can the risk of cardiovascular illnesses among the French be only a third compared to the Americans, when they are doing exactly the opposite of what is recommended in America as a preventive? The highly astonished scientists had to admit that they had found several reasons for this. The French:

- take their time when they eat
- eat three times a day
- divide up their meals (three courses) and have a varied diet
- eat more fruit and vegetables, so more fibre and vitamins
- eat good fats (olive oil, sunflower oil, goose and duck fat as well as fish)
- drink wine regularly, especially red wine

Since the broadcast of the report about the 'French paradox', which resulted in a rise in wine and goose fat consumption in the USA, the investigations have been extended. It has been found that the ideal way to eat, which should be taken as an example, is the very way that has always been common in the Mediterranean region and which has influenced most of Southern France.

Does this mean that the French do not have to change their eating habits because of these international findings? It is true that the situation in France is satisfying, compared to America where it has assumed dramatic proportions, but it does not mean that the situation has not been deteriorating significantly for some time. In fact, statistics show that the average weight of young people has risen markedly in the last few years (roughly 15% within twenty years).

Two years ago *Le Quotidien du Médecin* referred in an article to a survey that had been carried out among young recruits. It turned out that 25% had a cholesterol level that was too high, whereas twenty years ago it had only been 5%.

The 'French paradox' does therefore not apply to the coming generation. And this is for a good reason: it is the first generation to deny its heritage and to have adopted completely different eating habits, under the powerful influence of advertising, by unreservedly taking the North American way of eating, famous for Coca-Cola and hamburgers, as its own.

Adults stick more to their conventional eating habits as they are deeply rooted in tradition. There is, though, unquestionably, a trend towards the modern way of eating which can be attributed to the change in life-style, the hyper-standardisation of the food industry and the influence of advertising.

If we analyse this way of eating, we find that it is exactly the same as the American way. This means that it is just as likely to be hyperglycaemic. Among the foods that people prefer to eat nowadays are:

- white flour in all its forms (white bread, pastries made with yeast dough, sandwiches, hot-dogs, pizza, biscuits, cakes, crackers, noodles, low-fibre wholegrain flour. . .)
- sugar in fruit juices and other sweet drinks (cola. . .), in sweets and especially in chocolate bars
- potatoes, mainly in their most harmful processed form: chips, crisps or in a savoury baked dish
- white rice, the Western variety, which has a glycaemic index that is much too high if it is cooked in a lot of water which is then thrown away. If rice is cooked in water, this means that the soluble starch dissolves. If this water is thrown away, as is customary in the West, the

fibre is removed and this leads to an increase in the glycaemic index. For this reason the Asians cleverly cook their rice in very little water so that nothing needs to be thrown away and all the fibre is kept.

In the past people ate vegetables from their gardens, even if it was just in soup. As a result, the corresponding fibre intake was on average 30g per person per day. Nowadays it is 17g, whereas at least 30g to 40g should be eaten daily.

The crux of the matter

As will be seen, the Montignac Method will help you achieve a balanced body-weight. However, it is not only aimed at weight reduction but has also set the additional goals to:

⇧ prevent cardiovascular diseases effectively

⇧ restore maximum vitality

⇧ make sure that good food is enjoyed and eaten in company (which should never have changed). Food should be first and foremost an experience that is enjoyed together!

The method recommended here is simple. It is a matter of following the general concept of the 'glycaemic index' when you eat. In Phase I this will have to be done especially thoroughly.

How long this phase lasts will depend on the person and their respective goals and it can take a month or even several months. This time will be required to change eating habits, i.e. giving up the bad habits and beginning the good ones (the choice of 'good' carbohydrates and fats). The body will be 'detoxed', so to speak, and certain metabolic functions (insulin secretion) will have few demands made on them so that normality is restored.

This phase is easy to bear since it contains no quantity restrictions. For those who regularly subscribe to reduced-calorie diets this will be cause for joy, as they will be able to start eating again and yet slim at last.

However, Phase I is selective in as far as certain foods are removed ('bad' carbohydrates) or eaten in a particular way and at a specific time of day.

These meals are varied and balanced, since they are rich in proteins, fibre, vitamins, minerals salts and trace elements. Normally no feeling of deprivation occurs in Phase I, since you eat until you have had enough, so avoiding feeling ravenously hungry. Every day the advantages of this new way of eating will be right in front of your eyes.

Three meals a day

As said before, the principle of eating three meals a day is of the utmost importance. This principle means that no meal is to be missed and snacking between meals should be avoided. There are generally those who are afraid they will put on weight and who miss a meal, especially lunch.

'Shall we go and have lunch?' a secretary asks her colleague.

'No,' the latter replies, 'I've been invited out to supper tonight. I must watch my waistline. . .'

This illustrates the huge mistake people make daily. As we read in the chapter about reduced-calorie diets, the best way to put on weight is to have nothing to eat!

When a meal is missed, the body suffers from a shortage, whereupon it goes on the defensive; at the next meal this then results in the storage of fat reserves. Moreover, the more lavish this meal is, the greater the formation of fat reserves.

The role of the three meals

When you get up in the morning, the stomach has, theoretically, been empty for at least eight or nine hours.

The first meal of the day, breakfast, should therefore be the most substantial. In the past this was the case. Nowadays it is the most neglected meal. For many people breakfast is restricted to a single cup of coffee or tea on an empty stomach, with nothing to eat.

This practice does, of course, have catastrophic effects on the metabolism. In many cases, the following excuse is heard for this behaviour: 'Apart from the fact that we haven't any time to eat in the morning, it's mainly because we're not hungry.'

The explanation for this is simple! If you are not hungry in the morning, it is simply because you already ate too much in the evening. (It is a kind of vicious circle.)

To rediscover the right eating rhythm again you should begin by reducing your evening meal perceptibly (or, if necessary, cutting it out completely; this seems to contradict what has just been said, but the problem here is quite different).

To continue the good work started by breakfast, we recommend a normal lunch, or at least one that is substantial enough.

Your evening meal should, on the other hand, be as light as possible and eaten without fail as early as possible before you go to bed. This is because the body builds up its reserves again during the night. Eating something in the evening will make you fatter than eating something in the morning or at lunchtime.

We will go into these three daytime meals again in more detail and will recommend what you should do and not do.

Unfortunately most people do it completely the other way around. In our modern way of life, the role of these three meals has been reversed:

- breakfast is usually missed altogether, or is a very light meal
- lunch is normal, but often just a light meal
- supper is always too substantial

These are the excuses that are generally made:

- in the morning we are not hungry and don't have enough time (as we already know)
- at lunchtime we're working (unless there is a business lunch)
- evenings are our only chance to unwind; the whole family is reunited and eating something good is particularly appreciated because we're hungry

When a television journalist who appears on breakfast television was asked how she managed to get up every morning at four o'clock, she replied, 'I just had to change my habits!' This, dear readers, is the only thing asked of you: to change your habits.

Thousands have done it already; there is no reason why you should not succeed as well. If you really want to, you will reach your goal. Success depends on how determined you are.

Breakfast

As mentioned already, breakfast should be substantial. Since this is the first step to a new feeling of vitality, we recommend you take sufficient time to introduce this new plan.

You need to get up fifteen or twenty minutes earlier. This should not be too hard for you, as your sleep will have been noticeably improved by the changes made in your eating habits, especially where supper is concerned.

First of all, vitamins.

Since vitamin intake is often very 'poor' or neglected altogether, care must be taken to provide the necessary balance again. You need to know that it is the lack of vitamins, or inadequate amounts of them, that plays an important role in the development of fatigue. This applies mainly to the vitamin B group and vitamin C. Some people probably think that all you have to do is buy them at the chemist's.

You should only do that if it is absolutely necessary, in other words if it cannot be done naturally. There are several reasons for this.

Firstly on principle. If we are content that modern food contains too few important nutrients, and we therefore fall back on the synthetic products of the pharmaceutical industry to restore the balance, we will not bring any pressure to bear on the food industry, which no longer takes nutrient content in food production into account at all, to change its behaviour.

If the air were so polluted in the morning that we were scarcely able to breathe, the simplest thing would probably be to issue the advice to wear a face-mask or to ask people to buy regular doses of oxygen, as is already done in Japan. Getting rid of the pollution would, of course, be simpler, but it might mean that potential markets were lost to crafty business people, which would really be a shame.

Regardless of the dosage, synthetic vitamins are also less well assimilated than the natural vitamins contained in food. This is because further sub-stances are contained in natural products that we do not know about exactly and which have the effect of improving absorption.

To meet the daily requirement of Vitamin B, you only need to take (dried) brewer's yeast, which is a completely natural product. It can be found in supermarkets, pharmacies and in specialist shops. A course of yeast tablets would be beneficial, to last at least as long as Phase I; after that, it would be a good idea to repeat the course every two months.

A plentiful intake of B vitamins not only counteracts fatigue (as has already been said) but also ensures strong fingernails and beautiful hair. Vitamin B also contains chromium, which has a regulating effect on hyperinsulinism.

Fruit and Vitamin C

You can start breakfast with fresh fruit juice (lemon, grapefruit or even oran-ge). Kiwi fruit can also be recommended, as it contains five times more Vit-amin C than an orange (and in a more concentrated form).

Freshly squeezed fruit juice should be drunk immediately, as any delay will cause a considerable loss of vitamins. We recommend you give up commer-cially produced fruit juice, even when it is pure, as it scarcely contains any vitamins. We emphasise again that all fruit *must* be eaten first, i.e. on an empty stomach, and we have already explained the reasons for this.

Apart from getting used to not eating fruit at the end of a meal, we recommend you start the meal with it, at least as far as breakfast is concerned.

After eating fruit, you should wait fifteen or twenty minutes before eating anything else, so that the fruit can pass into the small intestine and there will no longer be a danger of it being trapped in the stomach because more food has been eaten.

The guidelines are not so strict with fruit that has been cooked, since there is no risk of fermentation. This applies especially to unsweetened jam since it contains less Vitamin C.

Different types of breakfast

The main aim of Phase I is, of course, the loss of those excess pounds. But there is another goal, that of normalising the function of the pancreas.

It has been proved that the energy low in the late morning is triggered by a breakfast of white bread, sugar, honey or jam. The pancreas, which has been 'treated badly' for years, must recover to a certain extent in order to lose the hypersensitivity that manifests itself in hyperinsulinism. It is going to be allowed to take things easy for a while, to give it a chance to function normally. This is taken into account in all the following breakfast suggestions.

The carbohydrate breakfast

This should be given preferential treatment, especially when you have breakfast at home. There are no restrictions of quantity or combinations of any kind:

- 'good' carbohydrates:
  - O 100% wholegrain bread
  - O wholegrain muesli without sugar
  - O wholegrain cereal flakes
  - O fruit jam, sugar-free
- milk products:
  - O quark or curd cheese with 0% fat content or low-fat yoghurt (0% fat content means milk products made from skimmed milk)
- drinks:
  - O skimmed milk
  - O decaffeinated coffee

O weak tea

O soya milk

All types of fat (butter, margarine) and whole milk products are excluded from this breakfast.

'Good' carbohydrates

⇨ **100% wholegrain bread**

Although we advise against eating bread at both other meals (apart from the occasional exception), it should be an essential part of breakfast, to ensure a balanced food intake.

Bread, certainly, but not any kind of bread. Wholegrain bread is best of all, where the whole grains have been used. Not to be confused with the wholegrain bread which is described as such but which is not produced with the whole grain. It certainly contains most of the ingredients of the grain, but part of it has been removed, and it is difficult to know how much.

Some bakeries even mix white flour with their wholegrain bread, either to make it look better or because it is easier to work. It is therefore hard to find a real wholegrain loaf that is exclusively made of wholegrain flour.

As far as bran loaves are concerned, these simply consist of white flour, to which bran is added. The bran is supposed to have to be organically grown, but this very rarely happens with bran loaves from the baker. Normal bran is full of pesticides, insecticides and herbicides.

The problem is that the baker generally tends to mix only a small amount of bran with the bread when he is making it. This is not for reasons of cost but because it makes the process easier. We might be able to put up with bran loaves containing at least 20% bran, as they contain a lot of fibre, which lowers blood sugar, but they lack vitamins and mineral salts.

If there are no genuine 100% wholegrain loaves for sale at the baker's – which would not be surprising, as they are not always available – it would be better to have it delivered or even to make it yourself. (It is available in a toasted form, so that it can be stored for several months. The price is well below average and it is especially competitive since the bread is made from organically produced flour, mixed with a raising agent).

So what should we put on this genuine wholegrain bread?

There are various possibilities according to taste. You can spread it with quark or curd cheese with 0% fat content, or sugar-free jam or both together.

Sugar-free jam has nothing to do with reduced-sugar jam. This is basically to be avoided, since it has 10 to 15% less sugar at best. This means that the sugar content is 45% instead of 55%.

Sugar-free jam on the other hand consists of 100% fruit (cooked naturally in fruit juice), 0% sugar and pectin (soluble fibre). You can have it delivered or buy it in specialist shops.

When choosing quark or curd cheese (with or without jam) you must make sure they contain 0% fat.

Breakfast cereals

Popular breakfast cereals mainly consist of corn, cornflakes or puffed rice and are served up especially to children for breakfast. These products of American origin have of course generous amounts of sugar and caramel, even when they do not have honey and chocolate added as well. It goes without saying that they are all forbidden during the weight-loss phase.

Recommended breakfast cereals consist of wholegrain flakes, made naturally of organically grown wholegrain cereal. They do not contain any kind of sugar or caramel.

The types of muesli that contain walnuts, hazelnuts, almonds or raisins are allowed if you only want to lose a few pounds. If you are very overweight (more than ten kilos), you should give them up at once and only eat them again in Phase II.

Permitted breakfast cereals can be mixed with quark or curd cheese with 0% fat content, yoghurt or cold or warm milk (skimmed, of course).

So that the cereal flakes can be easily digested, you should chew them thoroughly and with a lot of saliva. Of course it would be best to make these cereals yourself, using suitable equipment. When the grains are freshly ground (coarsely or finely) they contain the most vitamins.

A breakfast exclusively composed of fruit (when you are on holiday somewhere exotic, for example), is also allowed. However, you should add one skimmed-milk product at least, to ensure an adequate intake of proteins and calcium.

Drinks

Apart from the fact that you should eat something for breakfast, it is also very important to drink a lot. After you get up, your body should take in as much fluid as possible.

⇨ **Coffee**

It is recommended that you give up coffee (at least in Phase I), as it can cause an increase in insulin secretion in certain susceptible people with an impaired pancreas function. However, some scientists are of the opinion that caffeine encourages fat reduction. It is true that in the past, because of the way it was made, decaffeinated coffee was more harmful than coffee with caffeine. Today that is no longer the case.

Decaffeinated coffee can be drunk without moderation, especially as it tastes very good nowadays. Decaffeinated coffee is recommended for breakfast. Also, those of you who prefer milky coffee and can tolerate it do not need to give it up.

The claim that milky coffee has a harmful effect is completely unfounded. But there are certain cases where you should be advised against it; the deciding factor here is your personal physical make-up. Sometimes, because of an enzyme weakness, there is a milk intolerance that only really becomes obvious with a coffee/milk mixture, as the coffee alters the structure of the milk.

⇨ **Tea**

Although black tea has a small amount of caffeine it can be drunk without any hesitation. However, it should not be too strong. Tea has a remarkable diuretic effect; some people in Asia even claim that certain types of China tea can encourage weight reduction, but this has not been proved scientifically.

⇨ **Milk**

Skimmed milk is to be preferred, as wholemilk does not agree so well with adults. It also contains too many harmful saturated fats. Powdered skimmed milk is to be recommended, as it has a creamy consistency when water is added.

⇨ **Sweeteners**

It is quite clear that refined white sugar must be crossed off the menu forever, especially at breakfast. It is not actually sugar itself but the taste of sugar that you have to do without in the future. This is achieved by a gradual reduction in sugar consumption. Someone once said: 'Coffee does not taste of anything without sugar.' Anyone who has already given up sugar in coffee completely would never dream of adding it again.

To reduce sugar consumption, you could resort to sweeteners like aspartame. There have already been lots of discussions about this, which culminated in a violent disagreement. Since the economic significance of aspartame is considerable, both its opponents (sugar manufacturers) and its supporters (aspartame manufacturers) have carried out investigations by the dozen, to prove either its harmful or beneficial effects. Eventually the digestibility of aspartame prevailed. Even though it has been found that aspartame is not harmful, we do not know what effect it will have after it has been taken for years. This problem exists with all chemical food additives. Who knows their long-term consequences for the body?

We would therefore recommend that you only make use of aspartame very sparingly and very briefly (so only when necessary). It should only be used while you make the transition from sugar and then gradually reduced or at least only used very sporadically.

The advantages of fructose have already been highlighted, because it is not carcinogenic, for one, and, secondly, has a low glycaemic index; it is recommended especially in the manufacture of desserts. However, it has been held responsible for encouraging an increase in triglycerides. In reality, this only applies to those people with a serious problem in this area or who ingest more than 100g daily, which is an enormous amount. As using the Montignac Method achieves a considerable reduction of triglycerides, fructose can be used in moderation when baking.

Table 5 Carbohydrate Breakfast

Recommended	Tolerated	Forbidden
fresh fruit juice	commercial wholegrain bread	white bread
fruit (eat 15 min. earlier)	bran bread	rusks
100% wholegrain bread	muesli	croissant
wholegrain cereals without sugar	crispbread	brioche
unsweetened jam	German brown rye bread / pumpernickel	milk bread
0% fat quark / curd cheese	wholegrain cereal without sugar	pain au chocolate
low fat yoghurt	stewed fruit, no sugar	madeleines
powdered skimmed milk	skimmed milk (not powered)	jam
decaffeinated coffee	tea	honey
		full fat curd cheese
		full fat yoghurt
		full-cream or semi-skimmed milk
		coffee
		cocoa

Table 6 Fruit Breakfast

Recommended	Tolerated	Forbidden
oranges	cherries	bananas
mandarins	hazelnuts	fruit salad
grapefruit	prunes	tinned fruit
kiwi fruit	dates	candied fruit
apples	dried fruit	grapes
pears		
mango		
strawberries		
raspberries		
blackberries		
figs		
apricots		
nectarines		
plums		

The salty lipoprotein breakfast

Another breakfast variant is to have meat, sausage, eggs, cheese, etc. In a way it is an English breakfast, but with an important difference: all carbohydrates, even the 'good' ones are excluded (no bread). Since this breakfast contains a considerable amount of saturated fatty acids it is absolutely forbidden for those whose cholesterol level is too high.

After this sort of breakfast a lunch with no lipids (fats) and based on 'good' carbohydrates is advisable. Fruit is good as a snack between meals. As a rule you have this sort of breakfast in a hotel, where there is normally an extensive breakfast buffet available. The same advice applies to drinks as in the carbohydrate breakfast. This breakfast should be supplemented with a skimmed milk product (milk, quark/curd cheese, yoghurt).

Table 7 Lipoprotein Breakfast

Recommended	Tolerated	Forbidden
scrambled eggs	fruit juice ¼ hour earlier	white bread
hard-boiled eggs		wholegrain bread
fried eggs		rusks
omelette		croissant
bacon		milk bread
chipolata sausages		pain au chocolate
raw ham		madeleines
cooked ham		jam
cheese		honey
		muesli
		coffee
skimmed or semi-skimmed milk	full-cream milk	cocoa
		fruit
decaffeinated coffee	tea	

Small snacks

Those who are in the habit of having something to nibble in the late afternoon are probably suffering from slight hypoglycaemia. Once you have used the recommendations from this chapter, which provide for foods that have a less glycaemic effect, this feeling of hunger should quickly disappear.

Those of you who still like to eat something in your work breaks should have some fruit, an apple, for example. As alternatives there are almonds, walnuts and hazelnuts (very rich in vitamins) or 100% wholegrain bread.

You can also make do with a piece of cheese (if possible, low-fat cheese). Nowadays some cheese portions come ready-packed, which you can take to work with you without any problem, and without causing any unpleasant smell. Another possibility would be a hard-boiled egg.

Lunch

One of the main aims of Phase I, the protection of the pancreas, must be remembered at lunchtime as well. As at breakfast there are no restrictions of any sort as far as quantity is concerned. You should eat as much as is needed to give you a feeling of fullness.

It will normally include

- starter
- main course with 'very good' carbohydrates (with a very low glycaemic index, like fresh vegetables, for example)
- cheese or yoghurt

No bread should be served.

Starter

Starters can include raw vegetables, meat, fish, eggs, mussels or shellfish.

⇨ **Raw vegetables**

Raw vegetables are preferable as they normally have a large amount of fibre, which is good for filling the stomach. Raw vegetables also contain mineral salts and vitamins, which are assimilated better in their raw state. Raw vegetables recommended are:

- tomatoes
- cucumber
- celery

- mushrooms
- green beans
- leeks
- palm hearts
- white or red cabbage
- cauliflower
- avocado
- broccoli
- artichokes
- pickled gherkins
- radish

Also, all salads:

- lettuce
- chicory
- lamb's lettuce
- dandelion
- endive
- cress

Raw vegetables can be prepared with normal vinaigrette, i.e. oil, vinegar, salt and pepper and perhaps a little mustard. Olive oil is best, if possible, since it prevents cardiovascular diseases.

Celery can be prepared with a remoulade sauce (mayonnaise). Equally, some light crème fraîche or, even better, some quark/curd cheese with 0% fat content can be served with the cucumber.

Ready-made mayonnaise and vinaigrettes should of course be crossed off the menu, as they contain sugar and other undesirable additives, like starch or various 'unwelcome' types of flour.

In restaurants some raw vegetables are available which are forbidden in Phase I. These include

- cooked carrots
- potatoes
- sweetcorn
- rice
- couscous

There are no objections to walnuts, hazelnuts or pine nuts in salads. Croutons, however, are absolutely forbidden.

⇨ **Fish**

Fish should be eaten at every opportunity. Moreover, the oilier the fish (sardines, herrings, mackerel, wild salmon) the more it helps to reduce the cholesterol and triglyceride levels and protect the vascular walls. Raw salmon prepared with olive oil, and which can be an ideal starter in a restaurant, is particularly recommended.

Other possible fish starters include:

- sardines (grilled, or if possible, in olive oil)
- mackerel
- herring (without the undesirable potatoes, of course)
- anchovies
- tuna
- shrimps
- scallops
- prawns and scampi
- crayfish and lobster
- crab
- caviar and lumpfish roe
- all molluscs

All fish-based pâtés (without a puff pastry case) are acceptable, provided they are 'home-made' and not manufactured commercially (which, unfortunately, is the case more and more frequently).

Commercially prepared pâtés and ready-made foods contain numerous additives; flour-based binders, starch or thickening agents, sugar in all its various forms (glucose syrup and other polydextroses) and the taste-booster monosodium glutamate.

Suppliers should be approached about this and asked to divulge the composition of their products. The more they are made aware of the problem, the more notice they will take of it.

⇨ **Sausage**

For several reasons a certain amount of caution should prevail where sausage is concerned. First of all, sausages contain a great deal of saturated fatty acids (dependent on the type of sausage and the way it is manufactured). Secondly, sausages from supermarkets contain numerous additives (nitrites). Above all, they are made with meat of doubtful origin. In general this means pork from intensive livestock farming. Sausage consumption should therefore be restricted and the quality should always be checked.

⇨ Eggs

Eggs that are fresh and come from traditional poultry farms have a slightly reddish-brown yolk. Their nutritional value is of particular importance, as they contain numerous vitamins (A, D, K, E, B8, B9, and B12). This vitamin content depends, of course, on the quality of the egg.

There are certainly saturated fats in eggs, but these are barely assimilated because of the lecithin present. This therefore reduces the cardiovascular risk, where hypercholesterolaemia exists. A variety of starters can be made from eggs: hard-boiled eggs, egg mayonnaise, omelettes, fried eggs. . .

⇨ Further variations

According to opportunity and the breadth of your imagination, you can put together a balanced mixture of several of the starters already listed. If you order a mixed hors d'oeuvres as a starter in a restaurant, you should make your wishes very clear to the waiter. If you are not careful, you might find rice or sweetcorn or croutons mixed in when you come to eat it. Be especially cautious with the famous salad with bacon bits, since it always contains less bacon and more croutons to make up for it (which are not wanted).

Other possible starters include cheese; this usually means warm goat's cheese, served on salad leaves. When you order it you should take care to see that toast is not included.

Another starter, pâté de foie gras (goose or duck pâté without puff pastry) was deliberately not listed in the 'sausage' section, since we are talking about a special dish. The nutritional value of pâté de foie gras (without puff pastry) is still not recognised, although this starter contains a large quantity of monounsaturated fats (fatty acids). Nevertheless, it is not unreservedly recommended in Phase I (especially not for those who want to lose a lot of weight), as it consists of carbohydrates and lipids.

Toast is forbidden in Phase I anyway.

⇨ Forbidden starters

You might think that everything that is not allowed will be forbidden. That's not so! There is such a wide variety of products that not everything can be listed. If you know the basic rules of the Method, you will have no difficulty in putting starters that are not on the list (exotic foods, for example) into the right categories. Usually all you have to do is compare them with similar dishes.

The same is true for the starters to be totally avoided. With the knowledge you have gained so far you will usually be able to make a list of forbidden dishes yourself.

Nevertheless, here is a list of most forbidden starters:

- vol-au-vents
- puff pastry, including pies made with puff pastry
- quiches and English-style pasties
- soufflés made with white flour
- pasta
- white rice
- refined semolina
- anything involving potatoes

Main course

As a rule, the main course consists of meat, poultry or fish. We recommend accompanying vegetables containing 'good' carbohydrates, i.e. with a glycaemic index below 35. This usually means fresh vegetables or dry legumes, which have a lot of fibre.

⇨ **Meat**

Apart from the fact that you should eat fish at every opportunity, we recommend you choose the leanest types of meat, to restrict the consumption of saturated fats as much as possible.

Beef, lamb and pork are fairly high in fat; veal is less so, but to make up for that it conceals other risks at the moment. In this respect, poultry is streets ahead. Even sliced duck breast has far fewer saturated fats and a large amount of unsaturated fats (the good ones), which is only bettered by poultry.

You should of course beware of stews and pot-roasts, since these dishes usually come with a sauce made with white flour. Fortunately this is no longer the case in better restaurants. Be careful with breaded cutlets too, since the flour and crumb coating is on our unwanted list of undesirable products. However there are no objections to a sauce béarnaise, provided it is 'home-made'.

⇨ **Fish**

There are no restrictions of any sort with fish; it should not, however, be coated in flour or breadcrumbs before being fried. In the restaurant, as always, you should ask how it will be cooked. We recommend you should only order boiled or grilled fish.

As with meat, you should beware of sauces. A mixture of lemon juice and natural olive oil, which contains, as we know, a large amount of vitamins, is still best.

When cooking fish at home, frozen fish is the best guarantee of freshness. One possibility might be pollack or cod fillet, cooked either in a simple fish stock with mixed herbs (one soup spoon to one litre of water) or, with a splash of olive oil, in a covered pan on a low heat.

⇨ **Accompanying vegetables**

When ordering a dish in a restaurant, you should automatically ask about the side dishes. In nine out of ten cases the waiter will say chips or sauté potatoes. If you ask about other accompaniments, he will say, 'rice or noodles'.

In the restaurant you should therefore insist on being served something different from the other guests. If you persist, as a rule it is possible to obtain green beans, spinach, cauliflower or even broccoli. If there really is nothing else, we advise you to switch to salad.

⇨ The following **vegetables** are recommended in Phase I:
- courgettes
- aubergines
- tomatoes
- broccoli
- spinach
- turnips
- peppers
- fennel
- celery
- sorrel
- green beans
- mushrooms
- salsify
- cabbage
- cauliflower
- pickled cabbage
- Brussels sprouts

This list is of course, not complete. . .

Now for the question to end all questions:

'Cheese or dessert?'

In Phase I you should be content with cheese, as a rule. People probably imagine that it is really hard to eat cheese without any bread. Yet it is just as easy as drinking coffee without sugar. Once you've actually done it, you ask yourself why on earth you waited so long.

One ploy, which will achieve this target without any transition period, is to eat the cheese with salad.

You can also replace bread by spreading a piece of hard cheese (Edam, for example) with soft cheese (curd cheese).

If you really want to lose weight, you will know that you should not eat too much curd cheese, even if it is 0% fat. In the whey of curd cheese there is a quantity of carbohydrates (galactose) not to be sneezed at; an excessive consumption of these can mean that increased insulin will be secreted after the meal with the danger that the fats just eaten will be stored as fat reserves.

Therefore, no more than 80 to 100g should be eaten. Drained curd cheese is also to be preferred to cheese that has had the whey stirred in (if possible).

In Phase I, however, you must give up desserts without exception, since there are hardly any which do not contain sugar or fructose. At home you can make yourself a sugarless meringue or an egg custard with no problem.

Light lunch

It may be that, for various reasons, you do not have the time to have a normal lunch. In the past people would fall back on a sandwich, which is now – at least in Phase I – forbidden. In Phase II it will be allowed now and again, provided it is made with 100% wholegrain bread.

Since it is important not to miss out a meal, a way for you to fortify yourself must now be found. There are several alternatives.

⇨ **Fruit**

All fruit is allowed, except for bananas, since they contain far too many carbohydrates (glycaemic index 60). You can have three or four apples or oranges, for example. Another possibility might be to eat two apples, 200g of shelled walnuts, hazelnuts or almonds and two yoghurts.

⇨ **Cheese**

Any cheese is suitable; it should, however, contain as little fat as possible and not smell too strong (in case it is eaten at the office, for example). Another possibility would be to eat 250g of quark/curd cheese with 0% fat content, mixed with some strawberries, raspberries or even kiwi fruit. Some fruits, including blackberries, do not necessarily have to be eaten on an empty stomach.

There is only a very slight risk that this fruit will ferment. You can eat it without any problem with 0% fat quark/curd cheese. In Phase II it is even allowed at the end of a normal meal (as will be seen later).

A further alternative would be to eat two or three hard-boiled eggs, made easier to digest with a small tomato added.

⇨ **Bread**

To do without bread at two main meals (if they contain fats) is a basic principle that must be observed without fail. Perhaps some of you are think that eating 100% wholegrain bread could have been allowed. Fair enough! How will you manage, though, to have 100% wholegrain bread available at all times when it is hardly ever to be found in a restaurant?

Even if it were 100% wholegrain bread, at a main meal bread is simply superfluous. It has the unpleasant ability to cause flatulence, giving you a feeling of heaviness that can make that well-known state of fatigue even worse.

In addition, the aim of Phase I is to spare the pancreas as much as possible. With a lipoprotein meal the slightest secretion of insulin – even if it were not enough for the formation of fat reserves, would act as a brake on weight loss. You certainly won't put on weight, but you won't lose any either. . .

⇨ **Wine**

Just as with bread, we advise against wine in Phase I, especially if you want to lose a lot of weight. If you just want to shift a few extra pounds, you can have a maximum of a half a glass of wine at the end of the meal, preferably with cheese.

In Phase II we will deal in more detail with how wine should be drunk and when not to drink it.

In Phase I it would be better to drink water or tea. If you have ever tried to drink tea with a normal meal, as the English did in the past, you will probably have found that it not only tastes good but that it has a most agreeable effect. Tea promotes good digestion, something that applies to all warm drinks. If you like drinking herb tea (without sugar) when you eat, you should certainly do so. All types of tea are very welcome!

The evening meal

Of all the meals, the evening one should be the lightest (as has been explained already). Unfortunately, people often make a real banquet out of it – either at home or, on certain occasions, away from home.

At home you can easily change your habits. Since breakfast will now be much more substantial and lunch no longer missed, supper will not need to be as ample as it was before.

At any event, supper can be organised using the same principles as lunch. However, you will need to restrict the quantity, and above all, the fat intake. Also, you must not eat any meat if it has already been part of lunch.

At home you can begin by making a good vegetable soup, like they used to in the old days, with leeks, celery, turnip, cabbage (no potatoes!), and then have a small omelette with salad afterwards. Supper is the meal that offers us most opportunity to return to traditions that have been lost, by serving up certain foods that are no longer used like pulses (lentils, dried beans, chick-peas or peas).

It is advisable to have a carbohydrate-protein supper three or four times a week (a supper mainly containing carbohydrates with a low or very low glycaemic index). In Phase I you need to be careful only to eat foods that have been cooked without fat.

For example, you could begin with a good vegetable soup (without potatoes or carrots), such as mushroom or tomato soup, prepared without any fat, of course. Lentils, dried beans, chick-peas or peas can be served with onions or a mushroom or tomato sauce.

Another possibility would be a meal of wholemeal noodles, rice or semolina (Italians use it in savoury dishes), finished off with vegetables or a fatless sauce. These meals have the advantage of containing vegetable proteins, fibre, Vitamin B and numerous mineral salts.

Pudding after a carbohydrate evening meal should consist of either 0% fat curd cheese/yoghurt (with sugar-free jam, perhaps) or cooked fruit. If necessary you can eat 100% wholegrain bread with this meal, but this can make it rather indigestible.

The same rules apply to drinks as at breakfast; water, weak tea or herb tea are recommended. Now and again a small glass of red wine is allowed.

If you have had a substantial lunch and would therefore prefer a light meal in the evening, you can have just fruit and a yoghurt, or muesli with a skimmed milk product.

Table 8 Lipoproteins - Phase I Foods
Carbohydrates with a very low glycaemic index

STARTERS

	Raw Foods	Fish	Sausage	Others
Recommended	asparagus	smoked salmon	German salami	Mozzarella
	tomatoes	marinated salmon	raw ham	warm goat's
	cucumber	sardines	cooked ham	cheese
	artichokes	mackerel	chipolata sausages	veal sweetbreads
	peppers	herring	pork sausage	snails
	celery	anchovies	brawn	omelettes
	mushrooms	tuna	brawn sausage	hard-boiled eggs
	green beans	cod roe	endive with bacon	scrambled eggs
	leeks	shrimps	bits	egg mayonnaise
	palm hearts	mussels	pâté (with no flour)	eggs in aspic
	cabbage	prawns	foie gras	fish soup
	cauliflower	scampi		
	gherkins	crayfish		
	avocado	lobster		
	bean sprouts	caviar		
	lettuce	cockles		
	chicory	mussels		
	lamb's lettuce	whelks		
	dandelion	crabs		
	endive	squid		
	cress	scallops		
	broccoli			
	radish			
	carrots			
	Forbidden	**Avoid**	**Avoid**	**Forbidden**
	turnip		veal sausage	puff pastry
	corn		dumplings	vol-au-vents
	rice		flour-based pies	quiches
	potatoes			pancakes
				soufflés
				blinis
				toast
				croutons
				pizza
				doughnuts
				cheese fondue

Table 9 Lipoproteins - Phase I Foods
Carbohydrates with a very low glycaemic index

MAIN DISHES

Fish	Meat	Poultry	Sausage/Game/Offal
salmon mackerel tuna sardines herring perch cod pollack sole flounder ling whitefish pike-perch barbel trout all sea and river fish	beef veal pork mutton lamb	chicken fowl capon guinea fowl turkey goose duck quail pheasant pigeon rabbit	hare wild rabbit venison wild boar frying sausage blood sausage ham ox heart ox tongue veal sweetbreads kidneys pig's trotters
Forbidden	**Avoid**	**Avoid**	**Avoid**
fish in breadcrumbs	pieces of fat	the skin	

(Recommended — down the left margin)

Table 10 ACCOMPANIMENTS

Recommended	Recommended	Forbidden
green beans broccoli aubergines courgettes spinach mushrooms salsify celery sorrel chicory turnips leeks lentils chick-peas	tomatoes onions peppers ratatouille cauliflower cabbage sauerkraut lettuce vegetable pâté (no potato) artichoke	cous cous dried beans chestnuts potatoes rice pasta

Table 11 Carbohydrate Proteins - Phase I Foods
High Fibre

	Starters	Main course	Pudding
'Good' carbohydrates as desired	vegetable soup mushroom soup tomato soup	lentils dried beans peas broad beans whole rice wholegrain spaghetti wholegrain semolina	0% fat quart/curd cheese skimmed milk yoghurt stewed fruit cooked fruit fruit jam, sugar-free
Recommended	without fats without potatoes without carrots	without fats, served with tomato or mushroom sauce or with accompanying vegetables	without fats without sugar

Table 12 various spices and ingredients

To be eaten...				
...without any restrictions			... in moderation	... forbidden
gherkins mixed pickles pickling onions vinaigrette (home-made) green olives black olives tapenade celery salt	oils: olive oil sunflower oil groundnut oil walnut oil hazelnut oil grapeseed oil lemon Parmesan Gruyere	parsley tarragon garlic onions shallots them bay cinnamon basil chives savory dill	mustard salt pepper mayonnaise béarnaise sauce hollandaise sauce creme fraîche sauce	potato starch corn starch tomato ketchup ready-made mayonnaise Béchamel sauce flour-based sauce sugar caramel palm oil liquid paraffin

Further recommendations

We are now coming to the end of the basic explanations that are necessary to complete Phase I. If you used to eat too much sugar before you started using our nutritional principles, if you were a great fan of sweets and cakes and ate a lot of white flour products, as well as potatoes, you will be able to lose four to five kilos in the first month.

Do not stop after this time, though, and return to your bad old eating habits. If you do so, it is extremely probable that you will quickly put those lost pounds back on again. It is this yo-yo effect hat you must avoid at all costs. After this first phase you will continue to slim, provided you take notice of these recommendations.

So you will continue to lose weight, but at varying rates. It can happen much faster with some people than with others. Apart from some highly-strung men or those who have to take medicine (some medicines encourage weight gain), experience shows that men often get results faster than women.

Overweight in men can almost always be attributed to hyperinsulinism. Women, on the other hand, are more strongly influenced by their hormones, which can also have an effect on their weight. This does not mean, though, that they will be any less successful in the mid or long term.

However, it has been found that a good many women make heavier weather of losing weight than others do. There can be four reasons for slower weight loss:

- anxiety; this can stimulate abnormal insulin secretion
- hormone fluctuations during puberty and the menopause
- in rare cases there are thyroid problems (underactive thyroid)
- for a good many women, their body can initially, at least, be resistant to losing weight, because of the numerous deprivations during radical diets. These deprivations have perhaps even caused an increase in fat cells

If you have had problems with your cholesterol levels up to now, you will no longer have to worry about them in the future. Experience has shown that eating carbohydrates with a low glycaemic index in combination with good fats will in most cases make blood cholesterol levels normal. Above all, you should avoid saturated fats, which raise cholesterol levels (cholesterolaemia), and, instead, choose fats that reduce the bad cholesterol and increase the good one.

Although it is unlikely, your doctor might not happen to agree completely with this new eating method, since it doesn't fit with what he learnt when he was a student. As in many other areas, it takes some time in medicine too for new ideas and discoveries to be accepted, even when irrefutable scientific facts are on the table.

At any rate there are *no contraindications* when you follow the principles of this method. What sort of a risk could be hidden anyway in wholefoods with large amounts of fibre and micronutrients (vitamins, minerals salts, trace elements), which our ancestors were eating for millions of years before us?

Surely people won't claim that it is healthier to eat carbohydrates with a high glycaemic index (sugar, low-fibre flour, potatoes, modern high-yield varieties, industrially modified products)? A statement like that would be as ridiculous as the view that the polluted air of a big city was 'healthier' than the pure mountain air of Snowdonia.

But do not get worked up about criticism of your new way of eating. The critics will be amazed soon enough at the results that will inevitably become apparent: weight loss, better cholesterol levels. If you follow the rules of Phase I, it is impossible not to succeed. If you do not succeed, or if you only lose weight very slowly, then you are doing something wrong.

In that case, you should write down everything you are eating in the course of the day for a little while. With the help of this list, and once you have reminded yourself again of all the principles, you will be certain to find out where the problem lies. Perhaps you are eating much too much yoghurt or quark, for example, or too much vegetable soup containing, according to what others say, only 'permitted' vegetables such as tomatoes, sorrel, leeks etc., but this proves to be wrong.

Be less trusting, and check all ingredients. Perhaps the famous vegetable soups will turn out to be coming from a can or a carton. If you look at the ingredients given on the packet more closely, you will be astonished to find that the contents include not just the permitted vegetables, but also many 'bad' carbohydrates like cornflour, sugar, dextrose and other thickening agents, such as modified starch.

So be suspicious! Even if nutritional principles can be easily changed, they do require some effort in the first Phase at least and – let us be honest – some sacrifices. Do not waste these sacrifices by being thoughtless.

But take care! If you have been on a reduced calorie diet recently, or are on one at the moment, do not start with this method too abruptly. Your body is still just ticking over and will remember the deprivations of the recent diet. If you suddenly have a much bigger food intake, your body might be inclined to form fat reserves (this won't automatically happen). There might, therefore, be a small risk that you put on one or two kilos before losing weight. To avoid this unnecessary new weight gain, you should count calories for a few days at the start of the new method and increase your allowance in stages every five days by 100 calories, until you have reached the point where you feel full normally.

If you have just been on a badly balanced reduced-calorie diet you might (just at the beginning of the method) not necessarily become lighter, but your shape might improve. You feel that you are getting slimmer even though the pointer on the scales is not moving downwards. The explanation is simple. You are building up muscle mass again. In reality you are losing fat in favour of muscle, which takes up less space than fat but is heavier.

If your food was very low in fibre in the past, you should increase your fibre intake in stages, so that your gut can get used to it. The flora in the gut will increasingly adjust so that the larger quantity of fibre (wholegrain products, pulses, fruit, vegetables, raw vegetables) can be well digested. Initially you may have some flatulence or mild abdominal pain or a very soft and frequent bowel movement.

How long does Phase I take?

At the close of this chapter you ask quite justifiably, 'How long must I follow Phase I?' This actually depends on many criteria. We could answer by saying that Phase I should last until you have shed your excess weight. Since the speed at which weight loss is achieved varies from individual to individual there is no universally valid rule.

There might be another rule which said that Phase I ends when you have reached your ideal weight. Instead of 'ideal weight' we would prefer to speak of a 'balanced weight'. This is a very individual concept that relates to a point after which the body stabilises its weight by itself without any further weight being gained.

If you have to lose ten to fifteen kilos, Phase I can last anything from several weeks to several months. If you are only four or five kilos overweight you might be tempted to end Phase I as soon as the pounds are off.

The predominant aim of Phase I is not just to get rid of your excess pounds but to balance pancreas function so that it can raise its tolerance level to glucose again. This will take two to three months.

So if you end Phase I too early, there will be a risk that your pancreas will not have been able to recover sufficiently, even though the pounds have disappeared.

Assuming you did not want to lose any weight at all and were only following the principles of the Method in order to improve your state of health physically and mentally, you would still be faced with the same problem. You should keep to Phase I as long as possible in order to harmonise all your metabolic and digestive functions once and for all.

The question about the length of Phase I really should hardly be asked, as the transition to Phase II does not happen from one day to the next but takes place gradually. You will also find that Phase I is not at all disagreeable, since there are no quantity restrictions. You may even feel so well in Phase I that you don't want it to come to an end.

Twelve basic principles of Phase I

1. Eat until full without restricting the amount you eat and without counting calories.
2. Eat three meals a day at fixed times and never miss a meal.
3. Avoid any kind of snacking between meals. A small snack is possible in the late afternoon if supper is lighter to compensate.
4. The daily food intake will not be necessarily balanced in every meal (between the main components carbohydrates, lipids, proteins) but will be reached over the three main meals.
5. Breakfast is based on 'low glycaemic index' carbohydrates with few or no fats.
6. Lunch contains proteins, lipids and carbohydrates that must have a very low glycaemic index (no higher than 35).
7. Supper is either like lunch, but lighter and with fewer fats,
8. or it is based on carbohydrates. If saturated fats are used, the glycaemic index of the carbohydrates must not exceed 35. If no saturated fats are included and the intake of mono- and polyunsaturated fats is reduced to the minimum, the glycaemic index of carbohydrates can be between 35 and 50.
9. The consumption of saturated fats (meat, fatty types of sausage, butter, wholemilk products) should be restricted in favour of fish oils and olive oil, sunflower oil...
10. Avoid drinks containing sugar.
11. Do not drink more than one glass of wine (10cl) or beer (20cl) per meal. Avoid too-strong coffee; change to decaffeinated coffee.
12. Allow time to eat. Chew thoroughly and avoid any kind of tension when eating.

Summary

During this first part, step by step, we have got to know two new categories of carbohydrates: the 'good' ones, which you can eat regardless, and the 'bad' ones, which you must track down systematically and avoid. They differ from each other in the quantity of glucose absorbed by the intestines, which depends on several criteria:

- fibre content
- protein content
- the cooking time that conditions the gelatinisation of the starch
- the possible industrial modification of the starch

As the flour is ground ever finer, the glycaemic index rises and with it the insulin reaction. This excessive rise encourages storage of the fats that have been ingested with the meal. The glycaemic index of potatoes rises along with cooking temperature (deep- or shallow-fat frying).

This applies to all foods that contain starch, including those which have a low glycaemic index. This is the case with lentils (GI = 22 to 30), which can have a glycaemic index of 60 to 70 if they are cooked for hours on end until they turn into a thick jelly-like mixture (as often happens in India).

As we have seen, the glycaemic index is a key concept of the Montignac Method: you become fatter (or obese) because you suffer from hyperinsulinism. You suffer from hyperinsulinism because glycaemia is much too high at the end of a meal. Hyperglycaemia affects us regularly, because the carbohydrates we have eaten have a glycaemic index that is much too high.

For half a century dieticians and other diet experts were on the wrong track. They emphasised the 'quantitative' aspect of food and advised people who were obese to restrict their calorie intake, whereas nowadays we know that it is the *qualitative* aspect that matters.

In the earlier chapters we have distinguished between 'good' and 'bad' carbohydrates. One type makes you thin, the other ones make you fat, by triggering different metabolic mechanisms. Equally, there are 'good' and 'bad' fats. Some (indirectly) raise the cholesterol level, others lower it.

Using the principles of the Montignac Method we can transform the metabolic disease of obesity. We can eat until we are full, providing we choose the right foods, and by doing so we can eliminate our excess pounds once and for all, improve the way we feel in general and get more enjoyment out of life.

Table 13 Menu Examples in Phase I

Balanced lunches including carbohydrates with a very low glycaemic index

tomato salad	cucumber salad
veal cutlet	cod fillet (tomato sauce)
green lentils	peas
cheese	yoghurt
❖	❖
radishes and butter	chicory salad with nuts
turkey cutlet	grilled minced steak
pureed chick peas	broccoli
cheese	yoghurt
❖	❖
tabouleh with quinoa	palm hearts
salmon fillet	pork chop
courgette gratin	pureed celery
cheese	yoghurt
❖	❖
leek vinaigrette	grated carrot
grilled kidneys	leg of lamb
salsify	dried white beans
cheese	yoghurt
❖	❖
sardines in oil	asparagus vinaigrette
chipolata sausages	grilled blood sausage
cabbage	cauliflower puree
cheese	yoghurt
❖	❖
frisée with diced bacon	bouillon (fat removed)
grilled chicken	vegetable casserole
broccoli	leeks and cabbage
cheese	yoghurt
❖	❖
smoked salmon	tuna in olive oil
duck breast	steak tartare
mushrooms with parsley	leaf salad
cheese salad	yoghurt
❖	❖
red cabbage	grated carrot
skate with capers	grilled salmon
green bean puree	spinach
cheese	yoghurt
❖	❖
tomatoes with Mozzarella	artichoke hearts in vinaigrette
grilled chicken	entrecote steak
green beans	aubergines
cheese	yoghurt

❖

Drinks: water, weak black tea, herb tea, 10cl wine or 20cl beer

Table 14 Examples of Balanced Evening Meals in Phase I
including carbohydrates with a very low glycaemic index

home-made lentil soup	fish soup
fried eggs	cooked ham
ratatouille	salad
1 yoghurt	cheese
❖	❖
soup with dried peas	artichoke vinaigrette
stuffed tomatoes	smoked salmon
leaf salad	
1 yoghurt	salad
❖	❖
onion soup	leek soup
tuna fish	chicken breast and mayonnaise
leaf salad	leaf salad
strained quark	cheese
❖	❖
chicory salad	asparagus
cucumber with low-fat crème fraîche	poached fish fillet
turkey fillet	spinach
tomato sauce with basil	
yoghurt	cheese

❖

Drinks: water, weak black tea, herb tea, 10cl wine or 20cl beer

Table 15 Carbohydrate supper (without fat, except olive oil)

home-made vegetable soup	home-made vegetable soup	grated carrot
wholegrain rice or wild rice	wholegrain spaghetti	chick peas with tomato
with tomatoes	with tomato	unsweetened apple
1 natural yoghurt	drained quark	puree
❖	❖	❖
lentils and onions	oven-baked tomato	mushroom soup
(skimmed quark sauce)	with parsley	
salad and lemon	dried beans	whole rice with tomato
	(non-fat quark sauce)	
1 skimmed milk yoghurt	1 natural yoghurt	non-fat yoghurt
❖	❖	❖
couscous (wholegrain)	cucumber salad	lentil soup
with vegetables (GI<50)	with pureed mushrooms	quinoa with tomato
(without meat or fat)	and aubergines	sauce
sauce (non-fat quark + harissa	filled with non-fat quark	
+ a few drops of flavouring)	1 non-fat yoghurt	baked apple

Special recommendations

Caution with sauces

Conventional sauces and roux have a white flour base. They should there-fore be avoided. Nouvelle Cuisine sauces are usually made from juices from roasts which are enhanced with a little crème fraîche (more or less low-fat). You can get almost the same result if you stir in 0% fat curd cheese instead.

All you need for white meat is a sauce made from low-fat crème fraîche or curd cheese with 0% fat and some well-flavoured mustard, heated gently and poured over the meat before serving. Sliced mushrooms can also be added.

Mushrooms are also good if you want a creamy sauce without using flour. You need a blender for this. Purée the mushrooms and mix with some meat juices. This is the best way to make a delicious sauce for rabbit or hare stew or Coq au vin.

The best way to use mushrooms

Mushrooms can play a very important role, as they contain a lot of fibre and vitamins. It is a great pity that they are not on the menu more often. They can be used as a main course, as a tasty accompaniment or as a salad, made with fresh mushrooms.

After blanching the fresh mushrooms, drain them well for a quarter of an hour. Then slice them and cook them lightly in a little olive oil. Add garlic and parsley before serving.

Things worth knowing about food storage. . .

Those of you who grew up in the country will certainly be able to remember how your mother or grandmother only picked the lettuce in the garden a few minutes before it was eaten. The same thing applies to broad beans, tomatoes and all food that is eaten raw. In those days people thought fruit and vegetables tasted better if they were picked as near as possible to being eaten. In this way they instinctively avoided a vitamin loss, which occurs when food is stored.

Nowadays foodstuffs contain far fewer vitamins than they used to; this can be attributed to intensive cultivation and the considerably longer time span between harvesting and consumption.

Intensively grown spinach (where the aim is to have a higher yield per hec-tare) contains between 40 and 50mg vitamin C in each 100g. After one day's transportation, the vitamin C content has been halved and is therefore only

25mg. If the spinach is then kept in the fridge for another two days, another third of the vitamin C will be lost, leaving just 16mg. Cooking finally reduces the vitamin C content by a further 50%. At best, the spinach on your plate will contain just 8mg of vitamin C.

In contrast, 100g spinach from your own vegetable garden will contain at least 70mg vitamin C when picked. If it is eaten on the same day, there will be 35mg vitamin C left, roughly four times the quantity in the other spinach.

The vitamin loss in salad is even more serious. In less than quarter of an hour it has already lost 30% of its vitamins, and as much as 48% within an hour. This is appalling when you think of the long journey the salad on your plate has already had (between two and five days), not to mention the salad packed in plastic, ready for use, which has absolutely no vitamins left at all, but which in most cases contains chemical substances instead, or even salmonella.

Numerous restaurants advertise the fact that they will freshly prepare fish or shellfish only after they have been ordered. Why can this not be introduced with salad as well?

According to experts, cauliflower loses 2% of its vitamins hourly. When it is cut up it loses 8% in quarter of an hour and as much as 18% of its vitamin content in an hour. This turns a kitchen knife into a dangerous weapon, but it is nothing compared to a grater, which is really merciless. The vitamin C content of grated red cabbage is reduced by 62% within two hours.

A grater is a real 'instrument of torture', since it increases the cut surface of the vegetable two-hundred-fold. Grating exposes red cabbage, celery and even radish to a speeded-up vitamin loss. It will take no effort to imagine the vitamin content of ready-prepared foods, not to mention the instant products to be found nowadays on the shelves of our self-service shops.

The vegetables served up in canteens, hospitals etc. will also have been prepared in advance (one or two days before), i.e. cut and grated. 'And the police are doing nothing,' a journalist, observing this, once joked.

Be careful how you cook

Cooking damages the vitamins as well. But, contrary to what you might expect, vitamin loss does not depend that much on a high temperature. If spinach is blanched, for example, (at about 65 degrees C), 90% of its vitamin C content will be destroyed, whereas at 95 degrees C, only 18% is lost.

The explanation is simple. The eternally 'voracious' enzymes, whose function it is to decompose non-living material, are particularly active in the temperature range between 50 to 65 degrees C, whereas they have been almost neutralised at 95 degrees C. This is why cooked foods keep longer than raw. According to investigations that have been mainly carried out in Germany, vegetables lose more vitamins (C, B, B2) when they are boiled than when they are steamed. The shorter the cooking period, the fewer the vitamins destroyed. It is therefore better to cook food in a pressure cooker than to simmer it on a low heat, as used to happen in the past. Progress sometimes has its good sides.

After boiling, most of the vitamins and mineral salts will be in the cooking water. It should therefore be used again, to make soup, for example, provided the vegetables are organic. If they are not, you should be careful, since, along with the important nutrients, there will also be some harmful substance in the cooking water (nitrites, insecticides, pesticides, heavy metals...).

Also, when vegetable fats are heated to over 170 degrees C (when you fry steak, for example), they are changed into saturated fats (comparable to the meat's), which can have a negative effect on the cholesterol level. In this connection, grilled dishes, which are cooked on a charcoal grill, have been criticised fiercely for some years by cancer researchers.

They have actually discovered that the burnt fats are transformed into benzapyrene, an extremely carcinogenic substance. You should therefore switch to a vertical grill device where the fat can drip without coming into contact with the fire.

Since the microwave conquered the world it has been the subject of some violent disagreements. Noone disputes its extremely practical advantages, especially where saving time is concerned. However, what are its exact effects on the 'insides' of the food it deals with? At the present time, we still do not know very much about it, as the results of investigations into this are inexact and contradictory.

But if you are aware of the basic principle of a microwave – and most microwave users are not – you really have to ask yourself what happens to the vitamins, especially if you know how extremely sensitive they are.

The principle of a microwave oven is that the microwaves agitate the water molecules contained in food and the resulting warmth is passed on through heat exchange. What effect does this violent process have on the vitamins? The first alarming observations on this topic can still not be taken as proof as they do not have sufficient scientific support as yet.

Several more years will probably pass before we know for certain whether microwaves are as dangerous as some people say they are. After all, it took several generations before it could be proved that horizontal barbecue grills that people have been using for ages can produce carcinogenic materials.

When in doubt, then, rather than cooking regularly with it you should use the microwave more to warm up things occasionally at mealtimes. For this reason we therefore advise against young mothers using the microwave to warm bottles of milk for their babies. This is especially so as the baby runs the risk of being seriously burned. This is because it is difficult to gauge the internal temperature of the liquid; it can be boiling hot, for example, whereas the outside of the bottle is still cold or lukewarm. You also need to know that the milk is not sterilised as it is warmed in the microwave oven, unlike with the conventional method.

Beware of bad fats

Certain so-called saturated fats can have a negative effect, as we know, on cardiovascular diseases. This applies to butter, cream and the fats contained in sausage and meat (beef, veal, pork, lamb). An excessive consumption of these foods can therefore lead to an increase in the cholesterol level.

There are, however, as we also know, other fats that act as a protection of the vascular walls: fish oils, olive oil, sunflower oil and also goose and duck fat. When you select your foods according to the rules in Phase I you should continually be concerned to create a balanced relationship between the various fats.

We also recommend that you restrict the consumption of meat and sausage to three times a week; once a week you could have blood sausage, for example, as it contains a lot of iron. You could have poultry twice to three times a week and eggs twice.

Examples of a good and bad fat balance:

⇨ **A good balance:**

starter:	cold sausage (e.g. salami)
main course:	fish
pudding:	cheese or yoghurt with a natural fat content

⇨ **A bad balance:**

starter:	ham or endive with fried bacon pieces
main course:	entrecote steak or veal cutlet
pudding:	cheese or cream cheese

On the other five days you should preferably eat fish. It would be best if supper were based on a carbohydrate meal three times. Then there would be ten meals (seven breakfasts and three evening meals) out of twenty-one in total that contained large amounts of 'good' carbohydrates and no fats.

Table 16 Phase I Meals on Two Days a Week

7.10 get up	freshly squeezed juice from 2 lemons; 2 kiwis	freshly squeezed grapefruit juice; 1 pear; 1 kiwi fruit
7.30 breakfast	muesli (no sugar) 2 non-fat yoghurts decaffeinated coffee 1 cup skimmed milk	100% wholegrain bread fruit jam unsweetened
12.30 lunch	marinated mushrooms salmon new season's vegetables cheese	raw cucumber, radish entrecote broccoli cheese
16.30 snack	1 apple	1 apple
20.00 supper	guinea fowl ratatouille salad full-fat yoghurt	vegetable soup wholegrain noodles with mushrooms non-fat yoghurt

Phase II: Stabilising your weight with the Montignac Method

Phase II of the Montignac Method begins once you have successfully mastered Phase I. Phase II will help the final stabilisation of your weight.

You have now really lost weight and we congratulate you. It is a wonderful sense of achievement for you to see that you can reduce your weight so simply that you feel totally well. Phase II will now help you to maintain your weight as well so that your success is not just a temporary one. Every weight-loss method that is not geared to the long-term is completely pointless and can even have negative effects, so you should take note of some important points:

- You should set yourself a realistic goal; it is better to strive for an achievable weight-loss rather than dream of one that will never happen. Your body weight should not fall below a BMI level of 20.
- You should not restrict your food any longer than necessary, as this causes frustration. As soon as you start eating normally again, however, the body takes its revenge as a rule by immediately laying down fat reserves. But, since the Montignac Method is selective and not restrictive, this will present no obstacle in its use.
- You should learn how to deal with emotional pressures. The change in eating habits will certainly lead to a satisfying loss of weight, but this can only be one aspect of a fundamental change in your way of life.
- You need to be clear in your mind about your attitude to food. Eating should not be an answer to stress (caused by boredom, anxiety or lack of love). Suitable psychotherapy can be included, if needed relaxation exercises or yoga provide alternative ways of dealing with stress.
- If you have started a sporting activity to speed up the normalisation of the insulin function, you should keep this exercise up.

The Montignac method makes weight stabilisation easier for several reasons:

- There are no restrictions as far as quantity is concerned. After the end of Phase I there will therefore be no 'yo-yo effect' (the body does not react by putting on weight as it has not experience any frustration).
- The change in eating habits which was undertaken in Phase I can be continued without stress: as there is a wider choice, a great variety of food may be eaten.

- There will be no problems with your attitude to food, as Phase I is very well tolerated and helps a feeling of physical well-being to develop. From an educative point of view the Method represents a genuine behavioural therapy.

- Those who have kept exactly to the recommendations of the previous chapters will already clearly be feeling the positive effects.

It should, however, be emphasised that the body might possibly defend itself against the change in eating habits. Since the body has developed a real dependence on 'bad' carbohydrates over the years, it won't give in easily. This dependence is comparable to alcohol or drug dependency; in these cases breaking the habit can mean withdrawal symptoms.

Since the body has been supplied with glucose from an external source for a long time, its own glucose production has no longer been necessary. As soon as hypoglycaemia occurs, eating something supplies the required amount of glucose to the body. It therefore has no reason to produce glucose itself in order to keep the blood sugar at normal level.

A reduction in carbohydrate intake results in a lower supply of glucose, so the body is forced to produce glucose itself through its fat reserves. The body may possibly refuse at first to produce its own glucose. The result is temporary hypoglycaemia, which manifests itself mainly in feelings of tiredness. You must on no account give in and eat something sweet (even for a short time)! This resistance to change in the way that you eat, which can occur in the body in the first few weeks of Phase I, is most noticeable among strong people who go in for sport. Here too it manifests itself in sudden tiredness. In less severe cases it is best to eat almonds or hazelnuts, as they contain many nutrients. If there is a more serious reduction in energy, dried fruit (figs or apricots) are recommended, as they contain 'good carbohydrates'.

The body will very quickly understand that there is nothing for it but to reactivate its natural functions and manufacture glucose itself from its own fat reserves. Those who have eaten too little for a long period of time and who get fat just at the sight of something sweet will perhaps have to expect a slight weight gain (two or three kilos at most), but this will only be very temporary.

It is quite normal for the body to go onto the defensive after suffering years of deprivation. When it suddenly has the necessary energy it had been continuously deprived of, the body tends to store fat reserves. However, this condition only lasts for a few days. On no account should you make the mistake of eating less again, because that would just make the situation even worse. At all costs you must persevere!

The body will soon gain confidence again very quickly and understand that this is all meant for the best. Within a few days you will not only have lost this additional extra weight but will also have succeeded in reaching your first targets. Those who have been on a strict calorie-controlled diet should gradually increase their calorie intake, bearing in mind the recommended foods. This will avoid too great an imbalance, which can often lead to a temporary weight gain; this is caused by a body which has been 'starved' and which is still reacting as it previously did to a reduced calorie intake.

You may also seem to be getting thinner initially although you are not losing any weight. This is because muscle bulk is underdeveloped because of low-calorie diets (lack of protein) and for the first few days (or sometimes even weeks) a transfer of fat occurs so that fats are broken down in order to build up muscle bulk again.

How long does Phase I of the Montignac method take?

What probably interests you, the reader, the most at the moment, is how long Phase I lasts. This depends entirely on how much weight you want to lose, your individual sensitivity and how consistently you follow the principles of Phase I.

In order to reach the main goal of Phase I – to normalise the function of the pancreas – enough time should be allowed (from a few weeks to several months) so that there is a permanent improvement in insulin function.

Phase II is simply the natural extension of Phase I. However, some exceptions are allowed in this phase, which must be dealt with appropriately.

The previous chapters were about giving up bad eating habits and acquiring good ones. This alteration in eating habits continues to apply in Phase II; there is simply a change in that certain principles can be applied more flexibly.

Let us now come to the individual daily meals, this time from the viewpoint of the weight stabilisation of Phase II.

Breakfast

As far as breakfast is concerned, almost the same recommendations apply as in Phase I. It should still be substantial and consist of 100% wholegrain bread or wholegrain cereal. If you are eating proper 100% wholegrain bread, you can eat it with butter or margarine as you wish. Perhaps, however, only croissants or brioche are available (when you're travelling or eating breakfast with business colleagues). If it is an exception and you enjoy eating what is on offer, you should just go ahead and help yourself.

If you have done the right things during Phase I, your pancreas should now be able to withstand hyperglycaemia without triggering an excessive release of insulin and the resulting hypoglycaemia. The late-afternoon energy slump should be a thing of the past.

Those who occasionally prefer the salty lipoprotein breakfast should continue to avoid eating bread with it; under no circumstances should you stop this routine. This is dealt with again in the section on lunch. However much you are able to tolerate exceptions in Phase II – like for example, eating croissants or brioches – you should never deviate from the habit of always having fruit or fruit juice before breakfast. Mistakes are different from exceptions.

Lunch

In exceptional circumstances (business meals, family celebrations...) you can now have an aperitif before lunch, which, as you know, was forbidden in Phase I.

Aperitifs

There are several important principles to bear in mind with aperitifs.

Firstly, the aperitif should contain as little alcohol as possible. Alcohol which has been fermented is therefore to be preferred and distilled alcohol to be avoided, as the latter cannot be absorbed so well by the body. You should, therefore, at all costs abstain from high-proof alcohol like whisky, gin, vodka etc. If you feel a need for this type of strong alcohol, it is a sign that you are in a continuous state of inebriation. This also explains why devotees of high-proof alcohol drink it neat and on an empty stomach.

Since they are more or less in a hypoglycaemic state, alcohol temporarily makes the blood-sugar level rise, which has a brief stimulating effect. A habit of this sort encourages the feelings of fatigue that frequently occur after meals. For this reason it is advisable to drink wine, champagne or something similar (sparkling Saumur, Crémant-style wine. . .).

We also approve of the habit of offering a fruity white wine as an aperitif, such as wines from Germany or Alsace, Sauternes, Montbazillac, Barsac, Loupiac and Sainte-Croix-du-Mont. However, the habit of mixing liqueurs with white wine or, even worse, champagne, as a way of disguising its mediocre quality should for ever more be a thing of the past. Kir should be forbidden (in all its variations), even if this would have displeased its inventor, now deceased – a cathedral canon from the city of Dijon (Kir), which gave the aperitif its name. As is well known, liqueurs contain sugar, which in combination with alcohol will always trigger hypoglycaemia. Incidentally, punch, port and Sangria are included here too. Liqueurs are therefore the best way of anaesthetising yourself for the rest of the day or evening.

A further important principle that must be heeded without fail is never to drink anything on an empty stomach except water. It is in fact usual to serve drinks first and only serve up food a long time after (assuming any food is ordered at all). The drinks on offer mostly consist of 'bad' carbohydrates. The most important principle, therefore, is never to drink alcohol on an empty stomach. If you don't stick to this, it will undoubtedly have a disastrous effect on your metabolism.

Before you drink any alcohol, you should therefore have something to eat, but not just anything. To avoid the alcohol going straight into your bloodstream, it is important to make sure beforehand that the stomach is closed off. This occurs with the help of a sphincter muscle (pylorus), which is found between the stomach and the beginning of the small intestine. Eating proteins and lipids, which are digested slowly, ensure that the stomach is closed off.

Before drinking any alcohol you can eat some cubes of cheese for example, or some slices of German salami – no other sausage should be eaten as they contain a lot of additives. This small meal, which stays in the stomach for a long time, helps to neutralise the alcohol to a certain extent, as it partially absorbs it. As the lipids line the stomach, they ensure that the absorption of the alcohol by the stomach wall is avoided, or at least reduced. For this reason it is also claimed that the effect of alcohol is weakened if you swallow a spoonful of olive oil before drinking.

Wine

According to Dr Maury, 'wine has let itself be confined in the ghetto of alcoholic drinks'. It is therefore unfortunate that in many cases synthetic sweetened fruit juices, which often have a worse effect on the metabolism, are often drunk in preference to wine.

If wine is drunk in moderation (about two to three glasses daily with meals) it is an exquisite drink, since it has anti-allergenic and bactericidal properties and promotes the digestion and good health. It also contains a large amount of trace elements.

As with aperitifs, it is not the wine itself that causes tiredness after meals, but the way in which it is drunk. In a restaurant, if no one has an aperitif, wine is usually brought and served straightaway. If you give into temptation and drink your wine, you will have to expect the same consequences as with an aperitif.

So you have two possibilities: you either wait until the food is served or you order something small to eat (cheese, sausage, olives), so that your stomach closes off. You should always have eaten your starter before you start drinking wine. The fuller the stomach is, the less will be the negative effect of the alcohol. For this reason it would be best not to indulge in your wine until the middle of the meal. If you follow this rule you will no longer feel tired after eating and you will also have no digestive problems.

The quantity of wine drunk should always relate to the food eaten. If you drink water as well, you risk diluting the wine, which will then be digested quicker, whereas otherwise it would be absorbed with the pulped food. This means that you have to decide between wine and water when you eat.

Bread

In Phase II as well it is desirable to do without bread for two main meals. Bread should be part of your breakfast, that's where it belongs. You can eat as much of it then as you like. Bread should be considered a special food; you can feel free to drive a hundred kilometres to get it or bake it yourself. At the other two meals of the day, however, bread is taboo.

Going without bread at two main meals is also part of the principle. If you have reached this goal in Phase I, whatever you do you should keep to it and not relapse (apart from exceptional cases).

Bread is like cigarettes. Once you've given them up you should not start again, or you know what will happen in the end. All of us know former smokers who haven't touched a cigarette for ages and who then gradually start smoking again. After a long period of abstinence, which has aroused general admiration, they will be seen one day with a big cigar (cigars have nothing to do with cigarettes, they tell themselves in excuse). Since they don't always have large cigars to hand, they fall back on small cigars to begin with, then cigarillos – until the day when there are no cigarillos available and they start to smoke cigarettes again. This is the beginning of another beginning.

When bread is eaten with a meal with a high fat content – even if it's 100% wholegrain bread – there is a feeling of fullness. It is easy to understand why: for example, you eat a rich meal, consisting of two starters, a main course, cheese and a sweet pudding. If the principles of the method are observed with regard to the combination of foods as well as the way wine is drunk, after the meal you will feel light as a feather: In spite of the quantity of food that has been eaten there will be no problems with digesting nor any feelings of tiredness. If you eat a piece of bread with a similarly rich meal, flatulence will occur and there will be digestive problems. You should not revert to your old habits for all the tea in China.

One habit really to be condemned is when (triggered by hypoglycaemia) people sit down at the table and fall on the bread, which they then perhaps spread with butter as well. If they also had a glass of wine or an aperitif beforehand on an empty stomach, they will have already lost 50% of their vitality for the rest of the day.

Exceptions

Dealing with food in the right way means that you are able to deal with your body weight (what you can achieve) and with any exceptional situations. Therefore if you apply the principles of the method with perseverance you can allow yourself to make an occasional exception, without this having a negative effect on your overall success. This exception, for example, could be a soufflé containing some white flour, or fresh pasta served as an accompaniment, or even a small bowl of white rice.

Usually these exceptions are made with a sweet dessert. This is because you can leave part of your starter or main course discreetly on your plate, but refusing a pudding outright – in which there can be both sugar and white flour – is not without problems. Once won't do any harm.

These exceptions, however, should not be allowed to get so out of hand that you gradually revert back to your old habits.

Those of you who particularly like eating potatoes and don't like to do without them should allow yourselves some occasionally. However, when you do so it is important – as with all foods that have a hyperglycaemic effect – to eat high-fibre foods as well, to limit the increase in blood-sugar levels. If you prefer eating chips now and again, on no account should you eat any meat with them. Instead eat them with salad. You can even make a whole meal out of them. In this way, any damage will be limited to a certain extent.

There is the same problem with carrots. If you're not happy to give them up, you can eat them now and again, provided you supplement them with a high-fibre food.

⇨ **In Phase I** only foods with a very low glycaemic index were allowed as an accompaniment (those which are low in glucose and high in fibre).

⇨ **In Phase II**, as an accompaniment to fish and meat, some foods are again allowed which have a somewhat higher glycaemic index (wholegrain rice, wholemeal spaghetties, lentils, dried beans. . .). Lentils with bacon or leg of lamb with beans, for example, can even be regarded as no deviation. Every now and again you can even allow yourself to make a big exception and have, say, an accompanying dish with a high glycaemic index (white rice, potatoes).

In Phase II, too, fruit should be eaten on an empty stomach. An exception can be made for red fruits (strawberries, raspberries, blackberries). It is quite all right to eat these fruits (perhaps with unsweetened whipped cream) at the end of a meal, since they cause no fermentation and therefore no problems with digestion.

Evening meal

The basic principles which were established in Phase I regarding the evening meal are still valid in Phase II. There is a difference, however, in that, from time to time, certain exceptions are permitted (instead of at lunchtime). This does not mean, though, that major deviations can be made at each main meal.

The basic rule says that exceptions must fit in well with each other from a time point of view. If there have been too many deviations from the rules on one day, there is the danger that this will lead to tiredness, exhaustion etc. again in the following twenty-four hours (something you are no longer used to), to say nothing of the inevitable weight gain.

Moreover, you should only consider making an exception if there is a real treat in store. All the bad confectionery (sweets, chocolate bars) are excluded right from the word go. An exception must always be a concession to quality or an example of a gastronomic culture. This might be a delicious butter croissant, say, made by a true master of his craft. On the other hand, you should always avoid inferior industrially produced goods.

From wholefood sandwich to wholefood snack

Those of you who have access to wholemeal bread can occasionally treat yourself to a sandwich with lean meat, smoked salmon or raw vegetables. The same thing applies to 'wholefood snacks' (pizza, cakes, rolls) that have been made from high-fibre flour and organically grown products.

Present-day snacks would basically be acceptable if the missing fibre, mineral salts and vitamins were put back in again and the sugar, as well as the mostly saturated fats and pesticide residues, were taken out. These modern wholefood snacks would then be an ideal combination of the old and new way of eating.

But however groundbreaking, natural and realistic this new method of eating is, there is still no reason to indulge in excessive behaviour. To have something to eat because you want to or are in the mood, without thinking about it at all, is a really irresponsible way to behave.

Equally, thinking exclusively about the quality or origin of your food should also be vetoed; that just means going from one extreme to the other. This new awareness of food does not require you to do all your shopping in the health food shop, since even they cannot give you any 100% guarantees. But it does not mean that you completely disregard the numerous advantages of our modern consumer society either. What this new awareness should do most of all is help you be more discriminating in your selection of food, with the health aspect at the forefront of your mind from now on.

Our physical state of health is determined by the quality of our food and the air. Just as we strive to improve our air quality, we should make our food as varied as possible, enjoy that food, rediscover the variety of tastes, look after our gastronomic culture and pay the homage due to the genuine natural produce of old mother earth.

Implementing Phase II

Phase II is more varied than Phase I and it is easier to carry it through, as the basic principles are not as strictly interpreted. The division into 'forbidden' and 'permitted' foods made in Phase I no longer applies; in Phase II everything is allowed, although you shouldn't overdo it. It must be clear, though, that this is not about taking up your old eating habits again as soon as you have achieved your aim of losing some weight successfully and recovering your vitality. In all probability, if you relapse, those lost pounds and the fatigue will come back again (same cause – same effect). This means that the basic principles of Phase I will always be valid, just interpreted more loosely.

In Phase I exceptions were not allowed; in Phase II exceptions will be made. Do bear in mind, however, that any exceptions must still be based on the principles of Phase I.

Strictly speaking, Phase II is a phase of qualified freedom; it should become a firm habit as soon as possible. Dealing properly with exceptions is an art in itself; there are, however, certain rules you can keep to. Exceptions can, for example, be divided into two groups: minor and major.

⇨ **Among the minor exceptions:**

- a glass of wine or champagne as an aperitif after you have eaten some cheese, salami or olives. . .
- two glasses of wine with a meal
- a pudding that contains fructose (mousse or fruit) or a pudding made of chocolate with a high cocoa content
- a dish made with 'good' carbohydrates with vegetable fats (a piece of fillet in olive oil and lentils, lean meat with dried beans)
- toast (made with 100% wholegrain bread) with pâté de foie gras (no puff pastry) or salmon
- one slice of 100% wholegrain bread with cheese

⇨ **Among the major exceptions:**

- one aperitif + three glasses of wine at the same meal
- a starter with a 'bad' carbohydrate (soufflé, quiche, puff pastry)

⇨ **Some 'very slight' exceptions:**

- a main course with a 'bad' carbohydrate (white rice, noodles, potatoes)
- a pudding with a 'bad carbohydrate' (sugar, white flour)

In general, anything goes, but you ought to know that minor exceptions are only dealt with by the body with relatively few problems if you have successfully completed Phase I. Major exceptions also do no harm normally, provided they do not happen too often. Anyway, the scales will show you if any corrections need to be made or not. If you notice a recent weight increase, this can have two causes. Either your pancreas is no longer functioning perfectly or too many exceptions are being made. With a bit of sound common sense, you can take the appropriate action.

Dealing properly with exceptions in practice is much simpler than doing it in theory. It will not just be a possible weight gain that will show that too many exceptions have been made. Normally, the level of your energy will be the best way to establish whether the number of exceptions is too great. As soon as you have gone too far, there will be an immediate effect on the body, so that you automatically take counter measures; to a certain extent, you act instinctively.

Basic rules of Phase II

1. Never make more than two minor exceptions in each meal.

⇨ For example:

acceptable:	_not acceptable:_
two glasses of wine	one aperitif
chocolate mousse	two glasses of wine
>70% cocoa	lentils and bacon

2. Never cook more than one meal with a minor exception daily. This means that one of the two meals in Phase I is expanded.

3. Never have more than one out of three meals with one major exception, or one out of four meals with one major and two minor exceptions.

⇨ For example:

meal with one major exception:	_meal with one major exception and one small exception:_
avocado	smoke salmon
pollack, broccoli	leg of lamb with beans
apple cake	cream puff
one glass wine	three glasses of wine

Stabilising your weight

Let us spend a bit more time on the theory behind Phase II.

In the preceding chapters we explained how the glycaemic total of a meal ('post-prandial glycaemia') might trigger the storage of fats consumed during that meal.

You will see from Figure 17 that there is a very high risk of weight gain (obesity) with meals that have a glycaemic total of between 65 and 100. This also explains the large number of obese people who eat foods with a high glycaemic index, such as sugar, 70; potatoes, 95; low-fat fibre flour, 85; corn-flakes, 85 etc.

If the glycaemic total of a meal is between 50 and 65, hyperglycaemia will be lower, but still high enough to involve a potential risk of weight gain. This situation applies to those people who do eat carbohydrates with a high glycaemic index (potatoes, white flour, sugar) but who also eat foods with a low glycaemic index (green vegetables, lentils, beans, chick peas, fruit, spaghetti

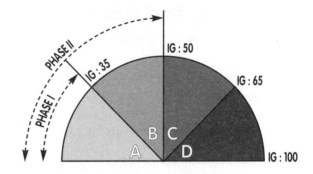

**Figure 17 Degree of risk of possible weight gain or
loss according to glycaemic total of meal**

Zone A: GI from 0 to 35: weight loss

Zone B: GI from 35 to 50: weight gain prevented

Zone C: GI from 50 to 65: risk of weight gain

Zone D: GI from 65 to 100: risk of major weight gain (obesity)

etc.) at the same time. As a result, the glycaemic total is slightly above the average but the risk of obesity is lower, or the obesity less pronounced. Overweight, worryingly, will often occur nevertheless.

If you want to slim down, the glycaemic total from your meal should not exceed 35, as we have seen. Only under these circumstances will insulin secretion (insulinaemia) be low enough to prevent the formation of fat reserves (lipogenesis) and stimulate the breakdown of fat reserves (lipolysis). We did this in Phase I, when we restricted ourselves to carbohydrates with a very low glycaemic index. In this way we were able to initiate weight loss without counting calories.

You could in fact stay in Phase I all your lives, without any problem, since the advice given to you would lead to a very nutritious way of eating. There are actually people who have felt so well in Phase I that they wanted to keep it up for ever. Even though Phase I will always remain a reference point for your way of eating, it can be criticised for excluding some foods which are usually on our menu. Phase I will certainly lead to a 'metabolic ideal', but it will restrict a normal social life and, especially, a gourmet life-style because of its rather dogmatic approach.

When people go on a reduced-calorie diet, a disrupted and increasingly hostile relationship with eating quickly develops, which in the worst cases can lead to anorexia. In contrast to this, the Montignac Method brings about a reconciliation with eating for us. But that is not all. The actual goal is to make you into a real gourmet (if you are not one already).

Eating: one of the most worthwhile things about being human

Cooking is a true art, like music or painting, accessible to everyone and symbolising that quality of life for which we all strive. To cultivate this art does not mean increasing our awareness just of the nutritional value of food but also of the culinary pleasure of discovering new kinds of food and different ways of preparing it. It would therefore be a pity to give up those foods forever that certainly do have critical effects on the metabolism, but which make up for it by their gastronomic importance.

It has never harmed anyone to eat an ice cream, a plate of potatoes or a piece of plum tart occasionally. But if you do that often, daily or even several times a day, you must not be surprised if there are undesirable side effects.

As Paracelsus once said, 'It is the dose (and its frequency) which determines the poison!'

In contrast to what you might mistakenly assume, the object of Phase II is not that you should regularly slip back into your old habits for a few days or weeks and then, having put on a few pounds again, repeat Phase I with renewed determination. The body will go along with this yo-yo effect three or four times, but will then become increasingly resistant, so that even Phase I is no longer as effective.

As we have already seen, there are exceptions in Phase II. If you want to go through Phase II without making any exceptions, there will be a wide-ranging spectrum of foods on offer, as you will now be able to eat carbohydrates with a glycaemic index up to 50.

You will be able to have basmati rice (GI = 50) with fish occasionally, for example, or drink orange juice (GI = 40), eat kidney beans (GI = 40) or even sweet potatoes (GI = 50). At mealtimes you can drink more than one glass of wine (two to three are possible) or even a whole beer (33cl) and still maintain your new weight. Your average glycaemia will certainly rise a little, but it will still be low enough to avoid a serious secretion of insulin and, with it, a new weight gain.

All other recommendations must continue to be followed, above all using the good fats (olive oils, fish oils) in preference to saturated fats, especially in the evening.

Exceptions can be made as well, making Phase II look much more diverse. This is how it differs fundamentally from all other diets. They lead you back to a wrong way of eating. The Montignac Method, however, offers you a genuine, constructive and positive alternative.

It is, therefore, possible to make exceptions and eat carbohydrates with a high glycaemic index, but only under certain conditions. That means that within the framework of a meal every food with a high glycaemic index *must* be balanced with its opposite. In other words, if you are going to have a food that increases the blood sugar level, like potatoes, you must eat something else with it that will lower the glycaemic total.

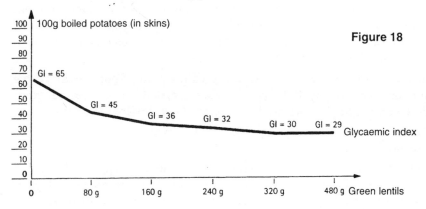

Development of a theoretical glycaemic result of a meal, consisting of 100g (unpeeled) boiled potatoes (GI = 65), depending on quantity of green lentils (GI = 22) eaten with them.

In the second half of the nineteenth century potato consumption rose sharply among the poorer sections of the population, especially among impoverished country people. Most of them ate potatoes every day but, in spite of this, they weren't fat. There is a simple explanation for this. For one thing, the potatoes eaten at that time were exclusively cooked in their skins in water or in the fire, leading to only a slight increase in the level of glycaemia (GI = 65), compared to chips or potato gratin (GI = 95). Secondly, potatoes were usually eaten then in a thick soup, containing numerous vegetables. So when they did eat potatoes (high GI) in those days they had a lot of carbohydrates with a very low glycaemic index at the same time. The glycaemic total was therefore moderate.

The Chinese, for instance, normally eat rice (carbohydrate with a high GI) with vegetables, which have a very low glycaemic index as a result of their high fibre content. The glycaemic total of their meal is therefore way below 50.

This is precisely what we are asking for in Phase II: regardless of what we eat, we must try to keep the glycaemic total of our meal as low as possible. This calculation can obviously never be absolutely exact. If we wanted more precise results, we would have to weigh the carbohydrates of all foods consumed and have a computer program analyse them together with all the other criteria. Experience, however, has shown that this is not really necessary, since people have also reached their goal just by applying some basic principles.

To understand these principles, we need to make some fundamental concepts clear.

We have suspected for some time that not all carbohydrate foods are the same. Some have high glycaemic figures like potatoes, others low ones like lentils. But you need to know that the pure carbohydrate content varies. For every 100g you find 55g of pure carbohydrate in bread (baguette), 33g in chips, 49g in crisps, 14g in unpeeled boiled potatoes, 17g in lentils, only 6g in cooked carrots and 5g in leaf salad or broccoli.

In order to compare like with like, a calculation of the glycaemic index of 'equal amounts of pure carbohydrate' was undertaken. Thus, the index obtained from the consumption of 100g sugar can be compared with that of 300g chips, 20g crisps, 588g lentils, 714g boiled potatoes or 2g salad. All these portions are comparable with regard to their glycaemic index, since they all tally on one point: they each contain 100g of pure carbohydrate.

As was said, the aim of Phase II is to balance out the exceptions. In practice this is complicated in that two criteria must be borne in mind:

- the glycaemic potential, measured by the glycaemic index
- the pure carbohydrate concentration of the food

The glycaemic index of carbohydrates

You know this concept well by now. To be able to differentiate between carbohydrates with a high glycaemic index and those with a low glycaemic index, you only need to take a look at Table 2 on page 00.

It is totally understandable that we sometimes fancy having something with a high glycaemic index. With the help of the table we can minimise the consequences. If we have boiled potatoes in their skins, for example, (GI = 65), this will not be too great a divergence. The slighter the effects of a divergence, the easier it will be to balance it out.

But as it is still a divergence, you will have to think about how this balancing out can be achieved. Common sense will tell you that it is difficult to bring the glycaemic total of a meal below 50 with a food that has a glycaemic index of 40 (kidney beans, for example).

You will therefore preferably need to use carbohydrates with a lower glycaemic index to achieve this balance. Logically, you might come to the conclusion that the lower the glycaemic index, the better this balance will be. You might also presume that those green vegetables with a glycaemic index of 15 would be ideal. In principle this would be correct, if the concentration of carbohydrates were the same. But we have seen above that it varies from one carbohydrate to the other. We need to explain this further.

Pure concentrations of carbohydrates

The glycaemic index of a food is important; however, it must correlate with the food's pure carbohydrate concentration. We also know that the amount of pure carbohydrate concentration in carbohydrate foods varies.

In accordance with traditional dietetics, carrots contain just as many carbohydrates as potatoes or lentils, for example. These carbohydrates differ, however, not only in their potential to cause glycaemia, but also in their concentration. There are already differences within food groups like potatoes, for example. Their glycaemic index varies according to the way they are cooked. Apart from these criteria, the pure carbohydrate concentration varies as well.

If the glycaemic index table is combined with that of the pure carbohydrate concentrations there will be both positive and negative results.

A surprisingly good result will be achieved by cooked carrots, which have a high glycaemic index but only a low concentration of pure carbohydrate, 6g per 100g, just a little higher than that of leaf salads. You can therefore assume that diverging with boiled carrots will have few glycaemic consequences. To achieve the same effects as with oven-baked potatoes, you would theoretically have to eat four or five times – or with chips six times – the quantity of carrots. You therefore have to eat 600g boiled carrots to trigger the same glycaemic total as with 100g chips.

You can therefore conclude from this that you will not have to beware of carrots as much in Phase II as you did in Phase I. If you find a few slices of this orange-coloured carbohydrate in a dish, you can enjoy it with a good conscience and not think about how to balance it out.

The same applies to all other carbohydrates with a high glycaemic index and low or very low concentration of pure carbohydrate, for example turnips, (3%), pumpkin (7%), water melon (7%), honeydew melon (6%) and beetroot (7%). If you do not eat these foods regularly, or in excessive quantities, you can allow them a certain degree of tolerance.

Unfortunately, those carbohydrates most suspect because of their very high glycaemic index will have a very negative impact, with chips at the top of the list. Of all the methods of preparing potatoes, chips not only have the highest glycaemic index (95) but the highest concentration of pure carbohydrate: 33g per 100g, i.e. 5.5 times more than boiled carrots, and 3.5 times more than potatoes boiled in their skins. Crisps are even worse than potatoes, as their concentration of pure carbohydrate is 49g per 100g, though their glycaemic index of 80 is somewhat lower.

Sugar comes off equally badly, which is no surprise. Its glycaemic index is high (70) and it has a maximum concentration of carbohydrate (100%), three times higher than chips and 16.6 times higher than carrots. You will therefore need roughly 140g lentils to compensate for 25g sugar and to lower the glycaemic total just to 50.

The last negative result concerns white flour products, which have a high concentration of pure carbohydrate (58% in very white bread, 55% in baguettes, 55% in semolina) as well as a high glycaemic index (70 for a baguette and 85 for hamburger buns). This also means that making exceptions with white bread and white flour products (pizza, sweet biscuits, cakes, crêpes, waffles...) will cost you dear, since it is very difficult to balance out largish amounts of them with the right carbohydrates.

Let us use an example to show what this balancing out might look like.

Let us imagine that your exception consists of one of those toasted sandwiches (GI = 85) you can get from railway cafés or motorway service stations. In order to compensate for 200g of this product, you would theoretically have to eat 682g of green lentils, and even then the glycaemic total would only drop to 53.

When you are on a journey, you will probably not have any lentils on hand to balance things out. On the motorway, the only compensating carbohydrates available are apples. The one disadvantage is that apples have a higher glycaemic index than lentils (30 instead of 22) and they contain fewer pure carbohydrates (12 compared to 17). To reduce your glycaemic total to just 57, you would theoretically have to eat 966g apples, which is almost impossible.

Fortunately, reality is not quite as alarming as theory, since other processes can contribute to the stabilisation of the glycaemic total. Carbohydrates with a low glycaemic index have been found to have a very much stronger balancing effect if they are eaten before the 'bad' carbohydrates. Therefore, in the example above, you should eat two or three apples first in order to trigger low glycaemia, and then your white bread sandwich. There will then be a much slighter increase in glycaemia.

Studies have confirmed this phenomenon. The increase in glycaemia result-ing from the consumption of a carbohydrate with a high glycaemic index has been shown to be much lower if that carbohydrate is eaten at the end of the meal. By virtue of this principle we can also establish that an exception made at the end of a meal (biscuits, bread with cheese, something sweet) will have less of an effect on the increase in the glycaemic total.

If on the other hand you begin the meal with an exception like potato salad, puff pastry, ravioli, crêpe or toast there will be a rapid and severe rise in glycaemia, and it will get harder and harder to achieve a balance with carbo-hydrates with a very low glycaemic index. To put it another way, the balanc-ing carbohydrates (lentils, salad, chick peas, soya beans, beans, green vege-tables, spaghetti al dente, quinoa, apples, pears…) will always have a much greater effect if they are eaten before any exceptions.

⇨ One of the main rules in Phase II is, therefore, that exceptions must be plan-ned beforehand. This is the only way to organise the balancing out in advance.

An example: It is Sunday. Many families tend to have a substantial meal at midday. Let us assume that you would like to have a piece of strawberry cake for pudding. This cake is an exception; as it contains both finely ground flour (GI = 85) and sugar (GI = 70). The hyperglycaemia triggered by their consumption is all the higher as white flour and sugar have a high pure carbohydrate concentration (58% and 100%).

To compensate for this exception, you therefore try to put together the rest of the meal using (exclusively) carbohydrates with a very low glycaemic index.

As a starter you should therefore choose raw vegetables and salad, for examp-le (tomatoes, cucumber, aubergines, mushrooms, lettuce cabbage, beansprouts, tabouleh made of quinoa…), which you know to have a very low glycaemic index. The accompaniments to the main dish should also be carbohydrates with a very low glycaemic index (broccoli, cauliflower, green beans and, es-pecially, green lentils). You will, of course, also have to go without bread, even wholegrain bread, since 100% wholegrain bread is rarely available and the wholegrain bread that is sold to you as such often has a glycaemic index of over 40.

Even if you drink three glasses of wine with this meal with an exception like strawberry cake at the end of it, the glycaemic total will be moderate and at any rate, low enough not to lead to any excessive insulin secretion.

But mind out! If you treat yourself to a helping of 'bad' carbohydrates with your meal, you should not just add 'good' carbohydrates to balance things out. You must not eat more to compensate for eating badly. If you eat a kilo of chips, it makes little sense to eat four kilos of salad beforehand to balance things out. Exceptions must be balanced out by helpings that must be changed according to their concentration of carbohydrates.

As we have already seen, the glycaemic index of boiled carrots and chips seems to be equally high, but the concentration of pure carbohydrate in chips is eight times higher. This means that if you have chips as an exception it should only ever be as a small or symbolic portion. You should be equally cautious with white flour and sugar, which as we have seen, tops the 'bad' carbohydrates along with chips and crisps, as they not only have a very high glycaemic index but also a very high carbohydrate concentration.

Even if we are running the risk of repeating ourselves, it is essential to plan any exception in advance, by thinking ahead about how to compensate for it. Never sit down at the table without knowing what you will be eating from beginning to end. If a big exception is part of your meal, at some point it may be too late to balance this out. This is why you must always know at the beginning of the meal what you expect to eat so that you can make your choice accordingly. Your exception may be a starter (e.g. something with puff pastry) or part of your main course (boiled peeled potatoes to go with your fish) or with your cheese (if you eat some bread with it) or a dessert.

It therefore does not make a great deal of sense to have the starter as one exception (crêpes or blinis), have another with your main course (mashed potato or polenta) and then finally to tell yourself when you have reached dessert, 'Now I must balance things out!' You have hardly any opportunity left to do so, unless you were to eat a kilo of green lentils or five kilos of salad, which is only a solution in theory. At any rate, the quantity of carbohydrates they contained would actually increase glycaemia.

You can see, therefore, that Phase II is a phase of freedom.

But this is a conditional or controlled freedom with principles that must become second nature to you. Thus, all exceptions are possible, provided you heed two basic principles:

- these exceptions must be out of the ordinary
- they must be balanced with regard to two criteria:
  - the glycaemic index
  - the pure carbohydrate concentration

Actually, you only need to take note of one basic principle: you should, above all, choose foods as exceptions that have low pure carbohydrate concentrations, since their glycaemic effect will be less and it is therefore relatively easy to balance them out. It can be very tempting to even out the extent of exceptions by differentiating between 'small' and 'big' exceptions and only paying any attention to the latter. You might consider, for example, having three glasses of wine with your meal or a small piece of white toast as a small exception, since they will only have slight repercussions on weight. However, the danger of this attitude is that you might play down these so-called small exceptions so much that they become a habit. It all mounts up; several small exceptions that are not balanced out can have the same damaging effects as a big exception. You must be aware of these small exceptions, as a matter of principle.

Another rule says you must never let yourself go even in the most difficult situations. As part of your social or business life, you may find yourself being served with a meal with three 'bad' carbohydrates, for example puff pastry as a starter, potatoes as an accompaniment to the main dish and a slice of cake with flour, butter and sugar as a pudding.

In such a critical situation you might persuade yourself that you had no other choice but to give in. But there are no situations where you do not have some room to manoeuvre and restrict the damage. If you are convinced by the Method (and after a successful Phase I, it would be surprising if you weren't), you should find it easy to resist.

Vegetarians, too, act out of personal conviction. They have decided not to eat any meat, and this is mostly respected by other people. Their conviction is usually so strong that they do not make any exceptions. Even when they are invited to spit-roasted lamb, they will eat none of it.

With the Montignac Method, the choice is never so stark; there is always some relative flexibility.

So if you do have puff pastry put down in front of you without warning, all you need to do is check the filling, so that you can eat the 'edible' ingredients and leave the rest on your plate. It would be surprising if you couldn't find some salad or even cheese. You can then make the cake an exception without too many scruples, avoiding the base and only eating the 'edible' filling. After the meal you should be aware that you have avoided a catastrophe, certainly, but that you have not been able to balance what you ate satisfactorily. Keep this information at the back of your mind so that you can organise your next meal especially carefully, sensibly following the basic principles of Phase I.

⇨ **Your scales will keep the real check on your weight.** There can be two reasons for putting on some weight: either your pancreas cannot tolerate the 'bad' carbohydrates yet and is reacting to the slightest rise in glycaemia, or you are making exceptions that are too big. You should take the right steps, that is, be particularly careful and repeat Phase I as often as possible.

There is, however, another indicator for the successful balancing of exceptions: your general well being. As soon as you have gone too far, you will very quickly notice that the negative side effects will reduce your vitality.

You will make the necessary adjustments, quite instinctively.

Table 17: Balancing Out Exceptions

Exceptions are printed in **bold**.
Balancing carbohydrates are in *italics*.

• *Lentil salad* with • vinaigrette (oil + vinegar) • veal cutlet • **white rice** • *leaf salad* • yoghurt	• *grated carrot* • cod • *green beans* • **crème brulée**	• *frisée salad with no croutons* • sausages • *dried pea puree* • **vanilla ice-cream**
• *spaghetti al dente* as a salad • **portion of pizza** • *leaf salad* • apple puree without sugar	• pâté de foie gras **+ 3 slices of toast** • duck breast • *ratatouille* • *leaf salad* • cheese	• 12 oysters **+ 2 slices of wholegrain rye bread** • marinated salmon • *leaf salad* • *chocolate mousse 70% cocoa*
• smoked salmon **+ *leaf salad*** • leg of lamb *flageolet beans* • **cheese** **+ 2 slices mixed flour bread**	• *vegetable soup*, (leeks, cabbage, celery, courgette) • omelette with sorrel • *leaf salad* • **crème caramel**	• leaf salad • *chilli* con carne • **plum cake**
• *leek* vinaigrette • *lentils* and bacon • **chocolate eclairs**	• *dried pea soup* • cooked ham • **mashed potato with olive oil** • *strawberries with no sugar*	• *artichoke hearts* • spaghetti al dente • sauce; creamed tofu with curry • **cheese cake**
• *spaghetti salad al dente* • pork chop • *green lentils* • cheese **+ 2 slices mixed flour bread**	• **melon** • buckwheat pancake with egg and ham • *leaf salad* • raspberries	• **water melon** • entrecote • *broccoli* • *fresh apricots poached in fructose*

Table 18 Average concentration
of pure carbohydrate per 100g carbohydrate foods

	Pure Carbohydrate	GI = Glycaem. Index
beer	5 g	110
potatoes baked in the oven	25 g	95
chips	33 g	95
puffed rice	85 g	95
instant potato powder	14 g	90
easy-cook rice	?? g	90
honey	80 g	90
cooked carrots	6 g	85
cornflakes	85 g	85
popcorn with no sugar	63 g	85
flour type 405 (white bread)	58 g	85
rice pudding	24 g	85
crisps	49 g	80
cooked broad beans	7 g	80
tapioca	94 g	80
crispbreads	60 g	80
pumpkin	7 g	75
flour type 505 (baguette)	55 g	75
water melon	7 g	75
flour type 605 (mixed flour bread)	53 g	70
sweetened cereals	80 g	70
chocolate bars (Mars)	60 g	70
peeled, boiled potatoes	20 g	70
sugar (sucrose)	100 g	70
turnip	3 g	70
cornstarch	88 g	70
corn	22 g	70
easy-cook long grain rice	24 g	70
cola drinks	11 g	70
pasta, ravioli	23 g	70
mixed flour bread type 805	50 g	65
boiled potatoes in their skins	14 g	65
white semolina	25 g	65
conventional jam	70 g	65
melon	6 g	65
banana	20 g	65
orange juice	11 g	65
raisins	66 g	65
white long grain rice	23 g	60
biscuits made with white flour	68 g	55
biscuits made with butter	75 g	55
white pasta, normal cooking time	23 g	55

Table 18 Average concentration
of pure carbohydrate per 100g carbohydrate foods

	Pure Carbohydrate	GI = Glycaem. Index
wholegrain bread (Type 1500)	47 g	50
buckwheat flour	65 g	50
buckwheat pancake	25 g	50
sweet potatoes	20 g	50
kiwi fruit	12 g	50
basmati rice	23 g	50
whole rice	23 g	50
sorbet	30 g	50
bran bread	40 g	45
bulgur (cooked)	25 g	45
black bread	45 g	40
fresh peas	10 g	40
grapes	16 g	40
squeezed orange juice	10 g	40
natural apple juice	17 g	40
wholegrain rye bread	49 g	40
wholegrain pasta (type 2000) 19g 40	19 g	40
kidney beans	11 g	40
fresh wholegrain bread (type 2000)	45 g	40
spaghetti al dente	25 g	35
ice-cream	25 g	35
fine Chinese noodles	15 g	35
original Indian corn	21 g	35
quinoa (cooked)	18 g	35
dried peas (cooked)	18 g	35
raw carrots	7 g	35
wholemilk yoghurt	4.5 g	35
skimmed milk yoghurt	5.3 g	35
orange	9 g	35
pear, fig	12 g	35
dried apricots	63 g	35
wholegrain pasta (type 2000)	17 g	30
milk (low-fat)	5 g	30
All-Bran	46 g	30
peach	9 g	30
apple	12 g	30
white beans	17 g	30
green beans	3 g	30
brown lentils	17 g	30
chick peas (cooked)	22 g	30
fruit spread with no additional sugar	37 g	30
dark chocolate 70% cocoa	57 g	22

Table 18 Average concentration
of pure carbohydrate per 100g carbohydrate foods

	Pure Carbohydrate	GI = Glycaem. Index
	17 g	22
green lentils	22 g	22
dried peas, unshelled (cooked)	17 g	22
cherries	10 g	22
plum, grapefruit	100 g	20
fructose	15 g	20
bean sprouts (cooked)	9 g	20
peanuts	10 g	20
fresh apricots	5 g	15
nuts	5 g	10
onions	28 g	10
garlic, green vegetables, lettuce, mushrooms, tomatoes, aubergines, peppers, cabbage, broccoli etc.	2-5 g	10

Table 19. Examples of Phase II meals

1st day

BREAKFAST
fruit
100% wholegrain bread + unsweetened
jam/marmalade
low-fat margarine
decaffeinated coffee
skimmed milk

LUNCH
avocado with vinaigrette sauce
steak with green beans
caramel cream
drink: 2 glasses of wine*

SUPPER
vegetable soup
mushroom omelette
lettuce
drained quark/curd cheese
drink: water

2nd day

BREAKFAST
orange juice
croissant + brioches**
butter
coffee + milk*

LUNCH
raw vegetables (tomato + cucumber)
grilled pollack fillet
spinach
cheese
drink: just one glass of wine

SUPPER
artichokes with vinaigrette sauce
scrambled egg and tomatoes
lettuce
drink: water

3rd day

BREAKFAST
Fruit
100% wholegrain bread
low-fat butter
decaffeinated coffee
skimmed milk

LUNCH
aperitif: diced cheese + 1 glass white
wine*
smoked salmon
leg of lamb with beans
lettuce
cheese
chocolate mousse
drink: 3 glasses of wine**

SUPPER
vegetable soup
stuffed tomatoes
lettuce
quark/curd cheese 0% fat
drink: water

4th day

BREAKFAST
scrambled eggs
bacon
sausage
coffee (decaffeinated) + milk

LUNCH
1 dozen oysters
grilled tuna with tomatoes
strawberry cake**
drink: 2 glasses of wine*

SUPPER
vegetable soup
cauliflower cheese
lettuce
yoghurt
drink: water

5th day
(major exception)
BREAKFAST
orange juice
cereals or quark/curd cheese
0%
coffee or decaffeinated coffee
+ skimmed milk

LUNCH
pâté de foie gras (no puff pastry
case)
grilled salmon + spinach
dark chocolate fondant**
drink: 3 glasses of wine**

SUPPER
cheese soufflé*
lentils with bacon*
cheese
meringue*
drink: 3 glasses of wine*

6th day
(complete return to Phase I)
BREAKFAST
100% wholegrain bread
quark/curd cheese 0% fat
coffee or decaffeinated coffee
+ skimmed milk

LUNCH
raw vegetables(cucumber,
mushrooms, radish)
poached pollack in tomato
sauce
cheese
drink: water, tea or herb tea

SUPPER
vegetable soup
cooked ham
lettuce
1 yoghurt

7th day
BREAKFAST
100% wholegrain bread
quark/curd cheese 0% fat+
unsweetened jam/marmalade
coffee or decaffeinated coffee
+ skimmed milk

LUNCH
chicory salad
entrecote and green beans
strawberries +unsweetened
whipped cream
drink: 1 glass wine

SUPPER
fruit:
1 orange, 1 apple, 1 pear
150g raspberries
drink: water

8th day
BREAKFAST
100% wholegrain bread
low-fat butter
coffee or decaffeinated coffee
+ skimmed milk

LUNCH
crab cocktail
tuna and aubergines
lettuce
cheese
drink: 2 glasses wine*

SUPPER
vegetable soup
lentils with vegetables
strawberries
drink: 1 glass wine

* = *minor exception*
** = *major exception*

Part Three

Important questions about our food

Do women eat differently?

Do women really eat differently? And if the answer is yes, do they need a different method to lose weight?

It is an interesting fact that women battle longer with overweight than men; this is to do with the way women's bodies are made. Because women have more fat cells (adipose tissue), they have a larger fat mass compared to men. It has been known for a long time that the size of fat cell increases in women (and men) who are obese. There is, however, also an increase in the number of fat cells, which is what makes obesity peculiar. It is possible to reduce the size of the fat cells, but not to decrease their number.

Investigations have now shown that it is the female body, above all, which will form new fat cells when its survival instinct is aroused by a reduced-calorie diet, a sign that there is a food shortage. Since this body has a greater potential for fat cells it is able to replace the lost pounds all the more quickly and increase weight in addition.

This makes women particularly keen to reach for the so-called protein drinks. But there is a big danger associated with these drinks: real complications can occur and in extreme cases an exaggerated diet of this type can even cause death. In the USA seventeen deaths have been registered that can be linked with an extreme reduced-calorie diet.

The women involved, who had had no previous symptoms, suffered from ventricular fibrillation and sudden cardiac arrest. In thirteen cases the proteins consumed were of a substandard quality. They contained only a little tryptophan and lacked the necessary calcium entirely. In the last four cases no plausible explanation could be found for their sudden deaths. One possible cause might have been the six-month duration of the diet, although it is not actually supposed to exceed four weeks.

Some women (and men, too) can suffer from depression when they become aware of their abnormal eating behaviour. In order to counteract depression and feelings of guilt, anorexia (the 'slimming illness') can develop; those affected have lost all feelings of hunger and manifest an extremely distorted relationship with food. Although no psychological disturbance was present initially, losing weight can become an obsession.

The young women who predominantly suffer from this disorder (they are usually no older than twenty-five) sometimes weigh less than forty kilos, which is why a stay in hospital and intensive treatment is often necessary to prevent them from dying. Unfortunately, the mortality rate (10%) is still far too high.

Puberty and eating

In the past, girls aged around eleven used to be thin, petite and even skinny. During puberty, which is accompanied by hormonal changes, the first feminine curves would become visible. Some became somewhat fatter and had spots on their faces. At seventeen, things had more or less settled down again. These young women possessed all the womanly attributes and had slim figures. When they were eighteen, their bodies had reached full maturity and a wasp waist emphasised a well-formed bust and behind. This was the age when they first experienced love and when they married.

Nowadays, a good many girls are already somewhat chubby before puberty. It's not really surprising, since their daily food consists of ravioli, white rice, potatoes, stuffed pancakes, quiches and pizzas from the deep-freeze, not to mention sweets, cakes, chocolate bars and sweet lemonade. Since their earliest childhood, their pancreas has been subjected to an excessive amount of strain.

During puberty, the way they eat becomes even worse (fast food, cola, sweet pastries, alcohol), which has a particularly detrimental effect at this stage. There will inevitably be some weight gain. To get rid of these extra pounds, meals are missed and reduced calorie diets are followed, with the visible negative results made worse by the fact that the body's reactions are especially sensitive during this stage of its development.

Typical repercussions will be:

- multiplication of fat cells (hyperplasia) because of reduction in food intake
- increased lack of nutrients, possibly leading to serious health problems: fatigue, anaemia, susceptibility to infection
- weight gain through the yo-yo effect, with possible disastrous effects on the psyche
- emergence of typical eating disorders: food cravings, followed by anorexia

Bulimia and anorexia

Although both these eating disorders seem to be complete opposites, they often alternate in young girls. These young girls begin by becoming dissatisfied with their appearance (35% cannot stand their bodies). Since the girls reject their outer appearance they concentrate on the current ideal of beauty and gradually restrict their food intake. This is the anorexic phase.

As soon as their natural hunger becomes overpowering, the girls develop a real compulsion to eat. This is the bulimic phase, which can be accompanied by deliberate vomiting and the taking of laxatives, diuretics or appetite suppressants.

This phase is particularly dangerous as it can lead to a decrease in calcium intake, which encourages palpitations and muscle weakness. Although clear successes have been achieved in the treatment of bulimia by making changes in the way people behave, the prospects are not as favourable with anorexia, although repeated treatments are given in hospital.

Does the Pill make you fat?

Almost 70% of young women aged between eighteen and twenty take the Pill. Unfortunately, the manufacturers remain silent about how much of an effect taking the Pill has on your weight.

Admittedly, there were weight changes with the first-generation contraceptive pills. However, nowadays people are convinced that modern (third generation) contraceptive pills no longer affect weight in any way, at least not for girls who are thin.

In the first half year of taking the Pill there may be at most a slight weight increase (about two kilos). This extra weight is not necessarily linked with an increased fat build-up; it is more likely that it is connected with increased water-retention because of the oestrogen in the Pill. If weight gain starts later, however, there will be a fat build-up, brought about by the anabolising effect of the progesterone.

However, investigations have shown that, even with third-generation Pills, there may be an increased release of insulin. Because of this, taking the pill may inevitably lead to an increase in metabolic disorders among overweight women who are already suffering from hyperinsulinism or insulin resistance. To make matters worse, doctors do not always prescribe a third-generation Pill with its minimal side effects right away, but carry on prescribing second-generation Pills.

A certain amount of caution is called for, therefore, especially with young women who are already overweight before they start taking the Pill. Some weight gain certainly cannot be ruled out. If there is a weight gain of more than three kilos, the doctor needs to be told. Particularly where the Pill is concerned, it is advisable to apply the principles of the Montignac Method, as this will lead to a decrease in insulin production.

One positive thing about the Pill is that it improves the condition of the skin (in acne); some versions are even especially suitable for the treatment of skin problems.

A beautiful skin – but how?

Your state of health can often be recognised by your skin, hair and fingernails. Pale skin, brittle hair with split ends, and split fingernails flecked with white are all indications that the body is lacking something. These problems can usually be attributed to an unbalanced diet, which has resulted in a lack of vitamins, trace elements, mineral salts, sulphur-containing amino acids and essential fatty acids:

- vitamins A and E are crucially important, for example, for the condition of the skin
- vitamin B_5 regulates the moisture content of the skin and strengthens the roots of the hair
- vitamin B_8 counteracts greasy hair and hair loss
- zinc regulates sebum secretion (increased with acne) and improves the hair structure

Various cosmetics in daily use do contain these micronutrients, but a diet rich in nutrients will always be the safest source of supply.

Taking synthetic supplements is not to be recommended, as they are badly absorbed in the gut. You can, however, supplement your diet with two natural products that are particularly rich in nutrients: wheat germ and brewer's yeast. Acne, which occurs during puberty, is linked with an increased secretion of sebum (excretion of fat by the skin) and can cause inflammation and infection. This skin disorder has no connection with diet. Teenage girls complaining about spots can carry on eating chocolate containing over 70% cocoa or sausage without worrying. Overexertion, lack of sleep and smoking can, however, visibly worsen the condition of the skin.

Women in their thirties

These are the best years of a woman's life; puberty is a distant memory and the menopause is still a long way ahead. At this stage in their lives, women are usually in the middle of their career; they are married (or in a stable relationship) and have children.

In this phase, between the ages of thirty and forty-five, women can be seen to differ in their eating habits. These differences depend on their education and, above all, on the time earmarked for preparing meals.

Investigations have shown that these eating habits lead on the whole to a sensitisation of the body, although this is not as bad as it is in puberty. Furthermore it has been found that women eat too much sugar, salt, white flour and too few vegetables, milk products etc., which can lead to shortages (lack of iron, vitamin C, E, B, calcium and magnesium). Many women suffer from overweight and cellulite, not to mention chronic fatigue. It is absolutely essential for these women who want to look good and be super fit to change the way they eat.

You should take care to:

- have an adequate magnesium intake
- have an adequate vitamin B6 and vitamin C intake
- avoid hypoglycaemia (low sugar level)

Slow weight loss

The rate at which men and women lose weight is not always the same. Even when they both have their meals together, eat exactly the same (type and quantity) and are also following the principles of the Method exactly, they can each lose a completely different amount of weight. For example, after a few months the man could have lost ten kilos, whereas the woman has only lost three.

The woman will now naturally think that the Montignac Method works better men than for women, forgetting that her best (female) friend (who advised her to buy the book) lost eight kilos without any problems within two months. She was perhaps a little overhasty in her conclusion. The explanation for the difference lies in the way individual factors affect weight loss. Sensitivity to a change in diet can vary between individual women, and there are also numerous differences between men and women.

Fat distribution: the difference between men and women

As we have said, women have a larger fat mass than men: 22 to 25%, compared to 17% in men. This difference can be attributed to a higher number of fat cells (adipose tissue). With women, the fat usually settles in the lower half of the body, possibly leading to cellulite. In men, the fat mass is more likely to be found in the upper half of the body.

This particular distribution of fat in women (upper thighs, hips, bottom) is used as an energy store in case of pregnancy or when breast-feeding. This function of building reserves, which was vital in the past to survive bad times (famines. . .) is hardly necessary nowadays in industrialised countries, but female bodies still possess this ancient reflex.

The fat cells in the lower half of the female body have special receptors, which, to a certain extent, are 'programmed' to form reserves. That is why weight will not be lost as fast in these areas of the body.

Increased sensitivity to hormones

Unlike men, women are at the mercy of hormonal fluctuations (puberty, menstruation, pregnancy, menopause) that can encourage weight gain. In some women, for example, an increase in appetite as well as a strong desire for something sweet can be noted a few days before menstruation. Many women also complain of mild depression at this time, which is linked with a lack of serotonin. The desire for something sweet helps to compensate for this lack. If certain hormone treatments are not carried out properly, this can also encourage weight gain.

A woman weighed down by her dieting past

In general men go on their first diet between the ages of thirty-five and forty-five at the earliest, when they make radical changes to their lifestyle. They not only want to lose weight, they take up sport again, stop smoking and make changes in their professional and sometimes even in their private lives. Since it is their first diet, their bodies react much better and weight loss is achieved faster.

Women, on the other hand, force themselves to go on a diet much earlier (from puberty) and much more often. They would like to be as slim as they were before puberty and live up to the ideals of slimness current in the magazines.

The years that follow are filled with reduced calorie diets. Because of the resulting fluctuations in weight (weight loss followed by new weight gain) certain regulatory mechanisms are set in motion in the body, which react to every new diet by forming fat reserves. Often there is even an increase in the fat cells so that as many reserves as possible can be laid down. This means that both hypertrophy (enlarged adipose tissue) and hyperplasia will be show themselves.

Caution – lack of protein!

Unlike men, women eat much smaller quantities of meat and cheese. Many women do not like eggs either. These eating habits mean that women often eat too little protein and this can even become a shortage when they are on a diet. However, if the protein content in the food eaten is too low, this will delay weight loss, because the fat mass will break down more slowly.

The effect of stress

As a result of some shattering event (death, divorce, unemployment) some women will lose weight. This is a kind of forced diet. These women simply cannot eat any more; it is as if their stomachs have been 'stapled', but this condition is usually only a temporary one. With stress a weight gain is more likely. In this case, behavioural and biochemical factors play a role.

Behavioural factors

Since the body is being subjected to serious strain, you start to eat to fill the alarming vacuum (the oral reflex gets going again).

There will be the following eating disorders:

- snacking repeatedly
- a strong desire for something sweet (to the point of addiction)
- attacks of bulimia

Forty percent of women also admit to eating just from boredom.

Biochemical factors

Stress triggers numerous biochemical reactions in the body:

- decrease in growth hormones
- release of endorphins
- release of hydrocortisone

These changes encourage lipogenesis (directly or through increased insulin secretion).

Women are more likely to put on weight than men, since they are more susceptible to stress. Because of the existing lack of nutrients (magnesium, vitamin B6, iron…) their bodies react particularly sensitively. However, stress can be reduced naturally by a change in eating habits.

Eating in pregnancy

Birth is a profound experience, which is why women should prepare for it both mentally and physically. Any necessary weight loss should always occur before pregnancy. However, most women tell themselves that there will be plenty of time for that after the birth of the baby, since they will be putting on weight during their pregnancy anyway. Wrong! If you are overweight, before your pregnancy is the time, if possible, to lose that weight, so that the excessive pounds do not 'settle' and complications with the foetus or mother (high blood pressure, diabetes, eclampsia) can be avoided.

In any event, we advise you against losing weight with the conventional method of dieting (reduced-calorie diet), since that would lead to a serious lack of vitamins, mineral salts and trace elements at the very time you need them most. However, if you lose weight according to the Montignac Method, you will be getting all the nutrients you need for the healthy growth of the baby through your food.

For nine months the mother-to-be must make sure that the foetus develops in the best possible way, but without depleting her own reserves. A nutritious supply of food is therefore recommended, to be divided equally throughout the day.

Alongside our basic principles, which meet the conditions above, the following recommendations should also be borne in mind:

- It is not necessary to eat for two. You should, however, eat particularly nutritious food.

- You should make sure you eat an adequate supply of animal proteins (meat, poultry, fish, eggs, milk products…) and vegetable proteins (wholegrain products, pulses, soya products), since they are essential for the baby's development. However, you should not eat liver more than once a week, to avoid the risk of damage from vitamin A.

- You should avoid eating raw meat (steak tartare, for example) and mussels (risk of infection); have as much calcium as possible to ensure strong bone formation for the baby without diminishing the mother's calcium reserves. For this reason, a milk product (milk, cheese, yoghurt, quark/curd cheese) should be eaten at every meal; preferably drink mineral water for an adequate supply of fluoride; be careful to have an adequate intake of iron to avoid anaemia, fatigue or susceptibility to infection (blood sausage, meat, pulses, dried fruit and eggs); have sufficient folic-acid to avoid deformities in the foetus. This can preferably be achieved by taking brewer's yeast, wheat germ and pulses; eat high-fibre foods, as they contain a lot of vitamins and mineral salts and help to prevent constipation. Fruit, raw vegetables, fresh vegetables, salad, bread, wholegrain cereals and pulses should therefore be a regular part of your eating plan; you should also make sure you have an adequate fluid intake to prevent dehydration, promote peristalsis (bowel function) and stop urine infections.

- You should, of course, give up alcohol to avoid putting the baby at risk. However, there are no objections to half a glass of red wine at the end of a meal, because the polyphenol contained in it improves the circulation of the blood.

- You should only take medicines or supplements on your doctor's advice.

- You should vary what you eat to avoid deficiencies and to accustom your child to a wide variety of food. After the fourth month of pregnancy the foetus has developed the ability to taste. If the baby has experienced different types of food in the womb, weaning will be easier.

- You should not smoke, as smokers often give birth to underweight babies.

A good many women put on a quite unjustifiable fifteen to twenty kilos during pregnancy. Normally there will be a weight increase of about eight kilos, which is made up as follows:

- foetus 3.5kg
- placenta 0.5kg
- womb 1.0kg
- amniotic fluid 0.7kg
- breast 1.0kg
- blood 1.3kg

The difference between the theoretical (eight kilos) and actual weight gain can be explained as follows: in the second three months of the pregnancy the foetus gains weight, but in the mother, because of an involuntary reflex, there can be a formation of fat deposits so that there are sufficient reserves in case of emergency. Eating foods that have a hyperglycaemic effect encourages this weight gain, which is why the Montignac Method is the best prevention.

However, sometimes the extra weight can be linked with excess fluid retention, which can lead to oedema, damaging blood circulation. In this case a doctor should be consulted, as this can sometimes conceal high blood pressure or albuminuria (protein in the urine). Your weight gain should always be in proportion with your initial weight and your height. A woman who is 1.50m tall and who weighs sixty kilos should not put on more than eight kilos during pregnancy.

A woman who is 1.75m tall but who only weighs fifty-two kilos can put on fifteen kilos without any problems, since her body has very few fat reserves. After giving birth she will quickly lose the excess pounds. Breast-feeding also encourages the fats to break down, so that she will soon be as slim as she was before her pregnancy.

Cellulite

All women find cellulite a nuisance but it only causes real concern when the symptoms become plainly visible. The best way of combating cellulite is to start preventing it as soon as possible. However, it is never too late to do something about it, even if there are no patent remedies. Nevertheless, the condition can be clearly improved if several measures are taken simultaneously.

Cellulite is a result of the following elements:

- natural predisposition
- hormone fluctuations
- bad eating habits
- unhealthy lifestyle

If something can be done about the last two, the development process can be halted and even reversed. But this improvement can only be brought about by a change in your whole way of life. The following steps should be taken:

⇧ Make an effort to reach your normal weight

Overweight makes cellulite worse. Those affected should try to lose weight so that the symptoms can be better recognised. Then the area of the cellulite itself can be treated.

⇧ Change your food

Above all, you should give up your bad eating habits.

⇧ Treat vein weakness

Vein weakness, generally described as 'bad circulation', is a common disorder that is invariably associated with cellulite. Circulatory disorders develop and are made worse by a sedentary way of life and our modern lifestyle (too-tight clothes, too-hot baths, too much sun).

Medical treatment can be very useful in serious cases, but usually old-fashioned household remedies (horse chestnut extract...) have proved most successful. They are just as effective as prescription medicines but have no side effects. These natural products are also available in every chemist's. A few minutes of keep-fit daily (skipping...) and some sporting activity two or three times a week (walking, jogging, cycling, swimming) are particularly recommended. Moreover, you should always use the stairs (two at a time) and never the lift.

⇧ Reduce stress

On no account should tranquillisers or any other anxiety-relieving medication be taken in order to reduce stress; instead you should use relaxation techniques or practise yoga. Acupuncture and homeopathic or herbal treatments are also suitable for stress management.

⇧ Use creams

Treating cellulite with special creams will only be successful if other steps are taken as well. A clear improvement in the surface of the skin has been shown after the application of creams with a caffeine basis, but these creams should not be massaged into the skin too much, to avoid a spread in the areas affected.

⇧ Miracle cures

There are in fact two miracle cures for cellulite, even though some people have found them to be totally ineffective. Breastfeeding is the first. Many readers have actually got rid of their cellulite by breastfeeding. However, they had also been applying the principles of the method, which had not been the case in earlier pregnancies.

Two factors were, therefore, necessary to achieve this success, breastfeeding and a simultaneous change in eating habits. Mothers-to-be might like to try it out. . .

For those of you who are not pregnant, cellulite can be combated with the second miracle cure by itself. This is a treatment involving cod-liver oil, together with a change in what you eat. It has been scientifically proved that the consumption of fish oils can lead to a clear reduction in the abdominal fat mass.

Some women have taken three spoonfuls of cod-liver oil daily over a period of at least four months and organised what they ate according to the principles of the method. The successes achieved ranged from an improvement of the cellulite to a complete disappearance of the orange-like dimples. However, you certainly need some courage to carry out this experiment and, most of all, you must keep it up!

The best thing to do is to pour the cod-liver oil into a glass (or a yoghurt pot that you then throw away), hold your nose and empty the glass in one go. . . Finally drink the juice of two lemons (without sugar, of course). It's hard, but it seems to work!

Medical treatment

If none of the measures listed above have a satisfactory conclusion, all that is left is a trip to the specialist, who will establish a suitable course of treatment (depending on the type of cellulite). At present there are numerous treatments possible: lymphatic drainage, mesotherapy... However, the disadvantage of these treatments is that they are very cost-intensive.

Water retention

It is necessary to make the distinction between overweight caused by an excessive fat mass and the extra weight that has been created by water retention.

Some women suffer from oedema, especially in the extremities, the abdominal area and the hands. This build-up of fluid depends in most cases on the menstrual cycle. Water retention is greatest before the start of a period and is characterised by tender breasts and a bloated stomach. Many of those affected also complain of fatigue, shortness of breath, headaches and constipation which can be accompanied by vein weakness, problems with water balance and an increased production of oestrogen.

What action can be taken?

⇧ Salt intake should be reduced to a minimum (5 to 8g per day) and you should therefore stop eating salty foods, such as sausage.

⇧ There should be an adequate supply of protein, which can be achieved by the consumption of fish, meat, eggs and cheese.

⇧ Care must be taken to ensure there is an adequate fluid intake, for water is the best diuretic. Women who complain about water retention generally have too small a fluid intake. The diuretic effect of water will be increased if the liquid is drunk when you are lying down, as is usual with water treatments at spas.

⇧ No diuretics should be taken since their effectiveness leaves a lot to be desired in most cases and the body very quickly gets used to them. Moreover, every time you stop taking them, the condition worsens.

⇧ Laxatives (to treat constipation) are also to be avoided. Normal bowel movement will be achieved solely by eating in a balanced way.

Circulatory disorders, however, need appropriate treatment. Preparations based on vitamin P (citrin or flavonoids) are particularly to be recommended. Other possible ways of treating this illness, which unfortunately can become chronic, include keeping the legs raised, giving up smoking and lymphatic drainage.

No smoking – no weight gain

According to statistics, stopping smoking very often leads to a weight gain. Unfortunately, this often acts a deterrent for many women.

Nowadays we know why smokers do not put on weight so quickly. Firstly, more energy is used up by smoking, as the basal metabolism is stimulated; secondly, peristalsis is speeded up which interferes with the absorption of nutrients, which are thus excreted through the gut. Nicotine also seems to inhibit the secretion of insulin.

During the difficult phase when you are breaking the habit you should not try to go on any reduced calorie diets, so as not to deprive yourself even further. The best way to avoid gaining weight is to use the Montignac Method.

Women around fifty

A hundred years ago a fifty-year-old woman was regarded as being old. Once she was no longer fertile and thus could no longer bear children the only role left for her was to be a grandmother. Today, a fifty-year-old woman is still young and there are enough means available to make sure she stays that way.

Hormone treatment (even if it is not absolutely necessary) can do a great deal to help you survive the menopause better and delay the ageing process. But staying young and preventing certain health risks (osteoporosis, cardiovascular diseases, cancer, weight gain) calls for a change in your eating habits. A balanced diet is what is required to stay beautiful, young and healthy, for you can be a grandmother and still have a youthful body.

The menopause

The menopause phase is particularly relevant as the majority of the female population are at this stage of their lives. This is the generation who were born during the baby boom in the period after the war. These women, who were the first to come into contact with the contraceptive pill, have a totally different attitude to the menopause than their mothers, who equated this phase with becoming old. Their daughters, however, merely see it as just another stage in their lives, since they know very well that the menopause (just like pregnancy) is not an illness but a natural process.

Up until thirty years ago, a doctor would only deal with a woman's physical concerns just before she became pregnant or if she was going to give birth. The introduction of the contraceptive pill changed all this and made a conversation with the doctor about contraception, gynaecological problems and sexuality an everyday occurrence. This made it possible to use medicines to treat the complaints that arise during the menopause.

What is the menopause?

During this phase, the sex hormones cease to function; the most obvious sign of this is the end of menstruation. The average age for this is around fifty, although there are differences according to race, climate and predisposition. The menopause usually starts at least two years earlier in smokers.

The Pill has made women aware that fertility and sexuality are two different things. They are not upset by the fact that they can no longer have children, as they know that this will not affect their sex lives.

The effects of the menopause

Once oestrogen production has stopped, there can be numerous problems that gradually appear:

- hot flushes
- incontinence
- dryness of the vagina (pain can be experienced during intercourse)
- dry skin and premature ageing
- the first signs of osteoporosis

- vascular disorders which can cause cardiovascular illnesses
- depression
- hormonal problems with possible weight gain

Many of these problems can be avoided by eating particular foods.

Staying slim during the menopause

This will depend on whether or not hormone treatment is being used.

⇧ No HRT

This is particularly tricky, as 44 % of those involved put on weight (four to six kilos). Practically no weight gain is seen among women who have always been slim. The reason why these women have never suffered from over-weight, in spite of their bad eating habits, is because of their robust pancreas. It is, therefore, unlikely that the pancreas will malfunction with the cessation of oestrogen, causing hyperinsulinism to occur. To make absolutely sure, these women only need to use the Montignac Method (Phase II).

There is more of a problem with women who are already fat, especially if they are considerably overweight. Of course, it would be better if their weight problem had been solved before the start of the menopause, since there will now be further weight gain. The fatter women are, the more weight they will put on, and vice-versa.

Table 20 Weight loss achieved
by women over 50 applying Phase I

BMI	Average weight loss after 4 months	Weight loss in %
24 to 29	– 9.2 kg	– 12.4 kg
30 and more	– 15.1 kg	– 16.8 kg

Source: Institut Vitalité et Nutrition

Experience has also shown that impressive results can be achieved by using the Montignac Method (especially when the principles of Phase I are followed exactly). Further weight gain can best avoided by a change in eating habits. However, all the factors that might have a negative effect on weight loss must be taken into account. This includes the points we have already listed and the factors to be mentioned at the end of the chapter.

⇧ On HRT

Even though weight gain occurs relatively often when no hormone treatment is used – the drop in oestrogen causes a worsening of hyperinsulinism – this does not mean that hormone treatments can work miracles. Their advantages certainly cannot be denied, but weight gain can by no means be ruled out, even though the statistical probability is less (31% compared with 44% of those not on HRT). This can be explained in the following way:

Oestrogens naturally encourage:
- an increase in the subcutaneous fat mass on the upper thighs
- abdominal lipolysis
- an increase in muscle mass (anabolising effect)
- water retention

Progestogens naturally encourage:
- the appetite
- an increase in abdominal fat mass (anabolising effect)
- an increase in muscle mass (anabolising effect)
- water retention

Potential weight gain can therefore be attributed to the following:
- a possible increase in fat mass
- a possible increase in muscle mass
- potential water retention

However, this potential weight gain depends on two criteria:
- existing excess weight (the fatter you are, the more likely you will be to put on weight)
- the prescribed method of treatment

Additional weight can be avoided if the correct hormone dosage is taken. If the treatment is carried out correctly, there will be no weight gain; on the contrary (*see* Table 21).

Table 21	Before treatment	After c. six months' hormone treatment
Average weight	51.7 ± 2.6 kg	56.8 ± 2.7 kg

The type of hormone, the dose prescribed and the precise way the dose is administered are, therefore, critically important. Unfortunately, doctors (and specialists, too, sometimes) all too often prescribe standard treatments without taking into account the individual needs of the woman concerned. It is quite clear that there can be no universally applicable hormone treatment for problems that can arise during the menopause. For this reason, each treatment should be based on individual criteria. However, many doctors seem to pay scarcely any attention to the aesthetic concerns of their patients. In the doctors' defence, the pharmaceutical industry can be said to bear a certain part of the blame, as they only mention the risk of gaining weight in very general terms so that it is not made clear how the hormones affect body weight when overweight already exists.

An unsuitable course of treatment can, therefore, trigger excess weight in any woman, especially in those who are already overweight. This means that hormone treatment must be constantly monitored, for at the slightest weight gain the treatment should be changed or even stopped completely.

As no details are given about how to avoid the risks of the treatment many women distance themselves from HRT treatment. This is also the reason why 30% of women do not take the hormones prescribed and 20% decide independently to stop taking the tablets within a year.

To avoid weight gain, the following measures should be taken when hormonal treatment for the menopause is used:

⇧ make sure that the treatment is suitable for your individual needs

⇧ use the Montignac Method to eliminate any additional risk of hyperinsulinism

Losing weight during the menopause

According to statistics, ten kilos of weight is gained on average between the ages of twenty and fifty. Pregnancies and bad eating habits have left their mark on numerous women. When they realise that there is a threat of further weight gain during the menopause (whether they are on HRT on not) they make a firm resolve to lose weight.

It is never too late to lose weight, but we can well imagine the frustrations suffered by those concerned (not to mention their disappointment at their failure) if they decide to tackle their excess pounds with the help of a reduced-calorie diet. Only by changing their eating habits can they achieve weight loss, and without depriving themselves of anything: this is particularly important during this phase, as woman are often prone to depression when their hormone levels drop.

Other factors during menopause

The menopause also encourages the development of other disorders:

- underactive thyroid
- depression
- stress caused by lifestyle changes
- lack of exercise

These problems can indirectly lead to weight gain.

Beware of depression!

During the menopause symptoms of fatigue can occur. If an underactive thyroid or iron deficiency can be ruled out as the cause, depression (connected directly or indirectly with the menopause) can be responsible. Professor A. Basdevant has investigated the effects of various psychological problems on body weight. From these it has been discovered that body weight can be influenced in either direction. According to predisposition, you put weight on or you lose it.

Table 22

Problems	Average weight gain		Average weight loss	
	Frequency	kg	Frequency	kg
depression	28%	+ 7.8 ± 4.3	27%	− 7.7 ± 3.6
death	9%	+ 8.5 ± 4.3	26%	− 6.7 ± 2.7
divorce	15%	+ 8.5 ± 4.3	36%	− 8.3 ± 4.2
family problems	14%	+ 6.9 ± 3.1	14%	− 6.6 ± 2.5
marriage problems	12%	+ 7.9 ± 3.1	12%	− 8 ± 3.7
sexual problems	15%	+ 9.5 ± 5.3	12%	− 7.8 ± 2.3
financial problems	10%	+ 7.1 ± 3.6	10%	− 6.3 ± 2.5
professional problems	14%	+ 8.2 ± 4.5	8%	− 6.5 ± 3.2
moving	2%	+ 5 ± 0.9	7%	− 5.6 ± 1.9

It is obvious from Table 22 that sexual problems trigger the greatest weight gain. They can also be accompanied by incontinence. It is clear from the survey into weight gain that an excess consumption of food (usually 'bad' carbohydrates) is often used to compensate for emotional problems. Moreover, the drop in hormone levels can also lead to an increased susceptibility to stress.

However, stress can encourage the secretion of hydrocortisone by the adrenal glands. This leads to:

- an increase in abdominal fat mass
- an increase in appetite
- raised water retention
- a reduction in muscle mass

These problems can be eliminated to a large degree with appropriate hormone treatment. Finally, care should be taken that there is an adequate intake of magnesium to increase the body's resistance.

Beware of acidosis!

Many doctors do not take the problem of acidosis seriously, as they are rarely faced with this problem. Nevertheless, it seems to occur increasingly often. You can see from the number of medications available in the USA without prescription that it needs to be taken seriously. In the opinion of Dr. Catherine Kousmine, the balance of acid bases in the body is of the utmost importance.

It is obvious from her first publications that the modern diet, which consists of highly processed foods with a glycaemic effect and too much meat, encourage acidosis to develop. The sympathetic nerve is triggered by acidosis and the following symptoms appear:

- fatigue, especially in the morning
- over-acidic gastric juices
- bloating
- constipation
- sensitivity to cold
- glucose intolerance
- irritability and increased susceptibility to stress

Dr Kousmine therefore recommends a reduction in the consumption of acid-forming foods (meat, tangy cheese, white bread, sugar, alcohol, tea, coffee) and that preference should be given to alkaline foods (egg yolk, yoghurt, fresh milk products, fresh vegetables, lemons, soya, fresh fruit, dried fruit) or neutral foods (walnuts, wholegrain cereals, real wholegrain bread). To counteract acidosis, you can also have freshly squeezed lemon juice (from two lemons) in the morning after getting up and alkalising water during the day.

If the condition is acute, good old sodium bicarbonate, which our grand-parents used to use, can still be helpful. All you have to do to check whether you suffer from acidosis or not is to buy the relevant litmus paper test strip in the chemist's and dip it in the first urine passed in the morning. The pH value should be over 7.

Women and constipation

By constipation we mean sluggish evacuation of the bowels together with dehydration (lack of fluid) of the bowel movement. This problem can be recognised by the absence of bowel movement (less than three times a week). With normal bowel function, evacuation of the bowel can occur anything between four times a week and three times a day.

Over half the population, three quarters of them women, complain about constipation. A distinction is made between two types of constipation:

- lack of urgency in emptying the bowels
- sluggish bowel function

Where there is a lack of urgency, medications and even diets are often totally ineffective. In severe cases, therefore, the problem should be eliminated by an exercise therapist who has the relevant knowledge.

Where the bowel is sluggish – the commonest type of constipation – treatment consists of:

⇧ changing to a balanced diet

⇧ normalising bowel function so that there are regular bowel movements even when no urge to evacuate is felt

⇧ physical exercise (walking, swimming, cycling, keep-fit) to strengthen the abdominal muscles

⇧ giving up laxatives, since they work against the body: if they are taken in excess they can cause bowel disease with persistent diarrhoea, abdominal pain and a marked reduction in calcium

⇧ giving up medications that cause constipation, such as antidepressants, for example

⇧ stopping reduced-calorie diets since they can affect stomach and bowel function

⇧ abandoning certain bad eating habits (taking liquid paraffin, for example), as they can become dangerous with time

Food and constipation

First of all, as soon as you get up, you should drink a glass of fresh fruit juice. Once the liquid reaches the empty stomach, stomach and bowel activity will be stimulated. Eating high-fibre foods is also recommended. This should particularly include wholegrain cereal (noodles, rice, 100% wholegrain bread. . .) and pulses, which contain large amounts of insoluble fibre. If required, 20g wheat bran (organically grown) can be used, stirred together with a milk product (quark/curd cheese, yoghurt).

A sudden increase in fibre intake can cause flatulence and abdominal pain, as the gut is still sensitive. For this reason the amount of wheat bran should be gradually increased. You can begin by taking 5g a day and increasing it by a further 5g every week until you reach the desired amount.

Even if the gut initially 'resists' a little, keep taking the bran, because these harmless 'protests' are an indication that bowel function is beginning to get back to normal. The recommendation is to take the necessary quantity of fibre exclusively through food and not to resort to vegetable flour, bulking agents or suppositories from the chemist's.

However, if the fluid intake is too low (less than 1.5 litres per day) constipation caused by hard bowel movements can become even worse. To encourage the emptying of the gall bladder and to counteract constipation, a tablespoon of olive oil is recommended after you get up. You can disguise the taste by having freshly squeezed lemon juice immediately afterwards.

Constipation should be treated without fail, in order to prevent the following disorders:

- reflux of gastric juices into the gullet
- hiatus hernia
- haemorrhoids
- varicose veins, resulting from abdominal pressure (during evacuation of the bowel)

Women and colitis

A hypersensitivity of the colon to the processes of fermentation and to fibre is usually involved with colitis (inflammation of the colon), spasms or irritation of the colon. The colon reacts with painful spasms or with inflammation of the lining of the colon. These disorders can be accompanied by constipation or diarrhoea.

When diverticulitis (spasms of the colon) is also present, the diet should contain fibre to avoid infection and to prevent cancer of the intestine. Where there is acute inflammation, fibre intake should be temporarily halted. In this case the following foods are permitted:

- lean meat with no sauce
- cooked ham with no rind or fat
- low-fat fish
- boiled eggs
- cheese (Emmenthal, Comté, Beaufort)
- white rice
- noodles
- semolina
- vegetable broth (made from sieved vegetables)
- cooked vegetables: cucumber, green beans
- pureed vegetables: broccoli, spinach, carrots, celery
- cooked fruit (peeled)
- fruit juice without pulp
- fruit jelly
- butter, oils, margarine
- mineral water (uncarbonated)

This unbalanced selection of foods should not form the basis of your diet for too long.

Where there are spasms of the colon (without diverticulitis) those affected tend to avoid more and more food because of the painful reactions of the bowels. This leads to drastic restrictions in diet and a completely unbalanced food intake. Many of those affected give up all milk products from the outset. However, this encourages calcium or protein deficiency, so for that reason this decision should not be taken too lightly. Also, allergies to milk proteins are very rare and can be detected using special allergy tests.

It is much more common to come across intolerance to lactose (sugar in milk), but this does not mean you have to stop eating soured milk (yoghurt, cheese), since these products are generally well tolerated. Furthermore, those affected tend on principle to avoid high-fibre foods. But they should not do this on any account, as fibre regulates disorders of the bowel function (diarrhoea or constipation). Fibre can be well tolerated if certain nutritional guidelines are observed.

During the first week there should be no fibre intake, so that the colon can start to recover. Then you should gradually start taking fibre in the form of tender fresh vegetables and peeled cooked fruit. In addition, you should have vitamin C in the form of fruit juice without pulp. Following that, you should gradually start eating raw vegetables again: vegetables, salad, fruit.

If required, bran can also be taken, in which case the bran intake can be increased by 5g a week until a total of 20g is reached. Wholegrain products are allowed as well.

Starch products should be thoroughly chewed so that the amylase of the saliva can be fully effective. Otherwise, the remnants of the starch would start to ferment in the colon in spite of the digestive enzymes from the pancreas and would cause flatulence, which can become very painful. Flatulence can be combated very effectively with charcoal or china clay. Antispasmodic medicines can be prescribed for severe pain.

It should also be remembered that flatulence can often be linked with eating too hastily. In such cases you should find somewhere quiet to eat and have your meal without rushing and in pleasant company. Those who eat alone tend to gobble down their food. You should also carry out breathing exercises several times a day; this strengthens the abdominal wall and 'massages the intestines' in an agreeable way. Ten minutes of relaxation after meals can also have a favourable effect.

Psychotherapeutic treatment of bowel disorders is only necessary if emotional problems are shown to be their cause. In normal cases, all that is needed is to adopt a healthy lifestyle, observe the nutritional guidelines and establish a good relationship between doctor and patient.

Women, Weight and age

The concept of old age may very well no longer be part of our world today, yet the saying, 'You can't deny your age,' has never been more relevant. In the eighteenth century you were already considered old by the time you were forty, especially as not even 4% of the population reached sixty. Nowadays people are technically 'old' in the administrative sense when they are sixty-five, but the current life expectancy for a woman is eighty-five.

Age, however, has nothing to do with how old you feel. Which of us doesn't know at least one woman who is still busy and active and amazingly sprightly at seventy or seventy-five?

The natural ageing process

Between the ages of sixty and seventy the body is subjected to a series of natural changes.

Physical changes

The weight of the organs and innards remains approximately the same, but there is a reduction in muscle mass. This reduction can be linked either to a decreased secretion of androgens (this causes reduced protein-building metabolism) or to a lack of exercise. This can have a disadvantageous effect on physical health, which can result in less mobility. There is a danger that people will only move between bed and chair, or, in the worst cases, become bed-ridden.

Although the fat mass in the abdominal area visibly increases, there is a tendency for subcutaneous fat to degenerate. There is also a decline in water balance by:

- 0.3 kilos yearly between the ages of sixty-five and seventy
- 0.7 kilos yearly after the age of seventy

This is popularly described as an old person 'drying up'.

Functional disorders

The ageing process in the body brings about the following changes in digestive functions:

- a change in the sense of taste caused by a shrinkage of the taste buds, which can be made worse by lack of zinc. 'Sweet' and 'salty' tastes are less pronounced. Food seems blander, and so people tend to use too much sugar, salt or spices
- dryness of the mouth caused by a shrinkage of the saliva glands or as a side-effect of certain medicines (containing atropine)
- chewing is affected by the state of the teeth/dentures
- increased reflux of food pulp by the duodenum in the stomach
- reduced secretion of gastric acids
- slower elimination from the stomach
- reduced secretion of pancreatic enzymes, making fats harder to digest
- decreased absorption of digested materials, which increases the lack of micronutrients: vitamins, mineral salts and trace elements
- increase of microbes because of sluggish bowel activity, which causes additional fermentation

Metabolic changes

These include:

- a slowing-down by 30% in protein renewal compared with young adults
- a rise in blood-sugar level after eating because of an inadequate insulin secretion, thus increasing the risk of insulin resistance
- increased sodium and water loss, which together with a decreased feeling of thirst heightens the risk of dehydration. Dehydration can be recognised if, when you pinch the skin, the fold in the skin remains. Taking diuretics or laxatives frequently will make the condition worse.

A changing way of life

The distinction here is between elderly women who spend their declining years in their own houses and those who go into a home.

⇨ Women living at home

There are two groups here:

- women who cook for themselves or have food provided by a family member or a home help. In this case they will have a relatively healthy and balanced diet
- women who have to make do with food that is delivered to their house

Many of these women are frequently widowed and feel alone and abandoned. They can feel depressed and disgruntled, and this can lead them to lose their appetite and retreat from the outside world. A vicious circle then ensues which can end with their being bedridden, unless steps are taken in time to prevent it. An excessive amount of medication can also often lead to lack of appetite, digestive problems and, in many cases, even to a loss of micronutrients.

⇨ Women who are living in an old people's home or a nursing home

- An old people's home has the advantage that food is ready prepared and eaten in company. The proviso is, however, that the women do not cut themselves off by staying in their rooms.
- In a nursing home, dieticians supervise the food.

Yet in reality the situation is not so rosy, as those advanced in years generally only eat what they like! Also, the meals are mostly cold and there are not enough staff to help those women who are no longer able to eat independently. Finally, there is no check to see whether the old people have actually eaten anything at all. Paradoxically it is those very (elderly) people in nursing homes who show clear symptoms of deficiencies, although they are under supervision and the food is being constantly checked.

Insufficient nutrition

Insufficient nutrition can occur when mistakes are repeatedly made in the diet. This can be shown by:
- fatigue or even apathy
- muscular atrophy
- weight loss (up to 15% of body weight)
- falls and broken bones
- mental confusion
- susceptibility to infection
- decreasing mental powers
- isolation
- disregard for certain nutritional guidelines
- poverty and alcohol consumption also make the condition worse

Conventional views are refuted

Old people need a large amount of nutrients and need to eat as much as adolescents, as intestinal absorption decreases and protein synthesis is sometimes affected. On no account should food intake be reduced just because you have reached a certain age, are no longer so active and make fewer demands. If food is reduced by a reduced-calorie diet, there will be a deficiency of micronutrients.

Old people require proteins and iron. There is therefore no need to restrict or even avoid meat consumption. Contrary to widespread opinion, eggs are not harmful to the liver and yoghurts will not cause a calcium deficiency. Both these foods should definitely be included on the menu for the elderly. It is equally not true that salt hardens the blood vessels, meat causes the formation of urea or pulses give rise to flatulence.

You should always eat well in order to live better and should therefore pay attention to:

⇧ calcium
⇧ vitamin D
⇧ vitamin B, B6, A, E and C
⇧ beware of diets as they can cause severe problems with kidney function
⇧ dangerously high blood pressure
⇧ progressive coronary diseases
⇧ serious forms of diabetes

Eating means sociability and pleasure

Food can only be called balanced if it is full of variety and takes taste and our preferences into account. Quality and presentation should therefore be of prime importance. To stimulate the appetite, it is recommended that you make mealtimes into real gourmet occasions.

But the way old people eat is determined most by the atmosphere, the surroundings and the community in which they live. Everyone knows that a meal taken in company tastes better. Food should therefore regain its hedonistic and Epicurean significance, which are of great importance. In the words of Brillat-Savarin: 'The pleasures of the table hold good at every age, in every situation, in every country and on every day; they can be combined with all other pleasures and at the end console us for the loss of those pleasures.'

And so we should always eat substantially and well.